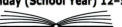

The
Whole
Tooth

*

ALSO BY MARVIN J. SCHISSEL, D.D.S.

Dentistry and Its Victims

The

How to Find a Good Dentist,

Whole

Keep Healthy Teeth, and Avoid the

Tooth

Incompetents, Quacks, and Frauds

＊

Marvin J. Schissel, D.D.S.,
and John E. Dodes, D.D.S.

St. Martin's Press
New York

Book design by Ellen R. Sasahara

Library of Congress Cataloging-in-Publication Data

Schissel, Marvin J.
    The whole tooth : how to find a good dentist, keep healthy teeth, and avoid the incompetents, quacks, and frauds / Marvin J. Schissel and John E. Dodes.—1st ed.
        p.   cm.
    Includes index.
    ISBN 0-312-15229-9
    1. Dentistry—Popular works.   2. Dental care—United States.
3. Quacks and quackery.   I. Dodes, John E.   II. Title.
RK61.S225   1997
617.6—dc20   96-27462
                                                              CIP

First Edition: March 1997

10 9 8 7 6 5 4 3 2

Note to Readers

The purpose of this book is to educate people about dentistry. While providing general guidance, it cannot take into account all the variables for any individual case, and so cannot be used to establish an appropriate diagnosis and treatment plan for a particular individual. This must be done by a competent qualified dentist.

Authors' Note

We tried to eliminate sexism from the book by the usual technique of using phrases like "he or she" and "his or her" and alternating pronouns, but this proved cumbersome and, we thought, disrupted the flow of language. So we stuck to the male pronoun exclusively, meaning it in the generic usage. Emphatically, every time we say "he," we mean "he or she," and every time we say "his," we mean "his or her," and every time we say "man" or "men," we also mean "woman" or "women." Emphatically.

Do not be angry with me if I tell you the truth.

—SOCRATES

Contents

✳

Part IV. Insurance and Managed Care

Part V. Conclusions

Preface

*

In the past twenty-five years, American dentistry has seen a great many changes, some for the better but many for the worse. Dental technology and marketing have enjoyed as well as suffered profound change, and so have the attitudes and traditions of practice. Long gone are the days when the choice of a dentist and the choice of treatment options were relatively simple. Today the dental consumer seeking the best deal is confronted by a profusion of bewildering alternatives: single practitioner, or union clinic, or insurance plan, or HMO, or referral scheme; fixed bridges or removable bridges or implants; conventional treatment or "alternative" approach, silver or plastic fillings, mouthwash rinses or gum surgery. Other questions arise: Is it safe to go to a dentist? Can I contract AIDS and hepatitis or other diseases from the dental office? Am I being poisoned by silver fillings, root canal treatments, or X rays? And, among the abundance of diagnostic techniques and treatments, which are the best? Which should I avoid?

These questions require candid answers, and so it is high time for an authoritative, up-to-date book for the dental consumer, union officials, HMO officers, insurance executives, legislators, and even dentists.

Among dentistry's problems are: economic factors that in too many situations dictate poor-quality treatment, the subsequent profusion of low-quality dentistry (Dr. Poorwork), and the disgraceful introduction and spread of quackery among dentists (Dr. Quack). This book contains an extensive section on quackery; in addition, whenever we describe a dental procedure, we try to show how differently it would be handled by Dr. Goodwork, Dr. Poorwork, or Dr. Quack.

In 1970 when Dr. Schissel's book *Dentistry and Its Victims* was first published, dentists were prohibited by the American Dental Association's (ADA) rules of ethics from telling a patient that his previous dentistry was poorly done. Shortly after the publication of Dr. Schissel's book the code was modified, but little has been accomplished in the direction of real consumer protection. It seems that a patient's greatest protection will come not from organized dentistry but from better information. We have attempted to illuminate areas of dental practice often kept secret.

The greatest change that all of us, doctors and patients, will experience will come from the restructuring of the way health care providers are reimbursed for their services. The section on managed care provides the necessary information to navigate the hazardous waters of third-party reimbursement schemes. This section also introduces Dr. Fraud, whose schemes and scams are milking billions of dollars from the dental reimbursement system.

The section on quackery was unnecessary thirty years ago; incompetence was a problem, but quackery was not. But today many dentists have succumbed to the economic temptation of quackery, and it is now widespread. Fraudulent dental care not only wastes economic resources but also can adversely affect one's health through misdiagnosis, unnecessary treatment, and the possible avoidance or delay of proper care.

The Glossary enables the reader to find any dental topic along with a short explanation. Glossary topics are examined in greater detail in the book.

We have been partners for more than eighteen years and have worked diligently to produce an accurate and up-to-date book on dentistry written with candor from the viewpoint of longtime consumer advocates. We could not have accomplished this book without the assistance of many of our dentist colleagues who shared with us their time and knowledge. We all hope that the public will be well served by this book.

Part I

*

Dentistry:
The Decaying
Profession

1. Introducing Dr. Poorwork and His Buddies, Dr. Quack and Dr. Fraud

*

W hen we graduated dental school many years ago, we were confident that there was a right way to do dentistry and that dental school had taught us this right way. Although at this early stage of our careers we were clumsy and slow in achieving good results, we had demonstrated on our school and state board licensing exams our ability to perform this right way. And we were confident that in time we would sharpen our skills and be able to perform good dentistry with increasing efficiency. We also assumed that all dentists treated their patients this right way. We were correct in all these assumptions—except for the last one.

As young dentists entering the real world of dental practice, we assumed that the careful, well-planned, and meticulously crafted dentistry we had been taught would be the standard for every dentist, but as we saw more and more of other dentists' work we soon realized that substandard dentistry was widespread. And the reason for this soon became clear to us—economics. Most distressing was that the victims, the patients receiving this substandard treatment, never suspected that the dentistry they had received was anything less than the best. The American Dental Association's historic conspiracy of silence had effectively done its job.

It's a shocking fact that, in the current economic climate, many American dentists actually *choose* to do bad work, and many others are forced into substandard practice by economic necessity. All bad dentists know how to do good work—all dentists have received similar training—but too often the economic context of practice permits bad dentistry to earn more money. In this book we call the typical bad dentist Dr. Poorwork. The villains of this book are all the Poorworks in the country, together with the dental societies and the profit-driven insurance industry, which are the machinery and the political expression of Poorwork privilege.

So the dental consumer has problems: how to judge whether a dentist is doing a good job, how to sift through and evaluate the torrent of information about mouth care, and where, if anywhere, to turn if a dentist is not providing excellent care. These are some of the problems this book addresses.

Among the health professions, dentistry is a particularly time-intensive field. The kind of quality that enables the patient to keep healthy teeth for a lifetime requires careful, meticulous attention to preventive and restorative programs, and this means taking adequate time. Speed is the death of good dentistry, so it is ironic that the fee-for-service tradition, which is the existing economic basis of compensation, rewards speed over quality. By way of illustration, take a routine dental task, a two-surface filling of moderate difficulty. It may take an experienced dentist half an hour to accomplish the meticulously prepared and finished filling that was taught in dental school, a filling that could be expected to last a generation or more (it would take a young, inexperienced dentist longer to do a decent job). Let us say that in a certain neighborhood the going fee is $50 a tooth surface ($100 for the two-surface filling). And let's assume that the average dental overhead is $150 per hour. So Dr. Goodwork, charging $100 for that half hour of work, gets to keep $25 after allowing for overhead. A dentist beset with financial pressures, or simply greedy, quickly realizes that if he does this filling in fifteen minutes, he doubles his receipts. He could even lower his fee to $80 for this procedure and still net more than Dr. Goodwork. As he gets more greedy, he'll do this type of filling in ten minutes, or even less. And so another Poorwork is born, competing successfully in the area of fee-per-service price.

The question may occur to some whether Poorwork's five-minute filling really is so much worse than Goodwork's fussy job. Absolutely. Later we go into this question in depth when we discuss various dental procedures and the different ways they would be handled by Goodwork and Poorwork.

Unfortunately, price has until recently been the only area where competition was allowed. Price could be advertised, but the ADA and state regulations did not permit Goodwork to claim superiority in quality, so he was in a no-win situation if he wanted to publicize his practice. Since discussions of quality were forbidden, the public tended to assume that all dentists were more or less equivalent in quality. So if Goodwork advertised, all he could say was, "Come to me and take advantage of my higher prices and slower work."

This was a travesty on the consumer. He was permitted to know what something costs but not what it was, and was thus prevented from having a real choice. Imagine a dealer in fine automobiles who is allowed to advertise the price of a car but not permitted to specify the make, model, age, or condition of the car. He is not allowed to claim that his cars are worth more, only that they *cost* more, which is not much of a selling point.

But as of June 14, 1996, a radical change in the advertising regulations has taken place in New York. The New York State Education Department, which regulates licensing and behavior of professionals, has approved new advertising rules for professionals that will permit testimonials, demonstrations, and even flamboyant fictional dramatizations. This will allow Dr. Poorwork to use the sorriest excesses of the advertising industry. We glumly anticipate seeing Dr. Poorwork's Aunt Nellie on the tube claiming that her perfect teeth resulted from Poorwork's great skill and compassion. But we doubt if Dr. Goodwork will be able to exploit the new rules since he will be bound by honesty.

Dr. Poorwork is the major villain of this book, but in a very real sense he is also a victim, in most cases a sad one. Most of the Poorworks we know are unhappy; they hate their work, and they hate their patients who are often uncomfortable and complaining. They often vent their frustrations on their staff, who in turn hate them. They never know the deep satisfaction of rescuing patients from pain and disability by quality care and of seeing these patients maintain continuing excellent oral health over the years. They never know the fulfillment of installing a carefully done, complex restoration that enables a dentally crippled patient to smile and eat again with comfort and efficiency. They never know the gratitude, loyalty, and appreciation of a family enjoying lifelong high-quality care. Instead of savoring the rewards of producing fine dentistry, Poorwork must contemplate the dreary daily routine of making hasty, sloppy fillings that are bound to fail prematurely, pulling teeth that ought to be restored, and coming up with lies and evasions for patients who want to know why they are in pain and their teeth are constantly breaking down. When he looks in the mirror he sees someone who is not doing the excellent job he was trained to do. Each time that Poorwork sees a patient, he knows that the best advice he could give that patient would be to go to another dentist. Because he has trouble keeping patients, he belongs to many union and insurance plans, which maintain his supply of patients. He may even resort to fraudulent reporting on insurance claim forms, because the "managed care" fees are so low he couldn't otherwise make a living. This adds another dimension to his wretched professional life: He now takes on an additional name, Dr. Fraud. Altogether, this adds up to a most miserable professional existence.

Why would anyone choose to travel this dismal path? The answer, as usual, is economics, complicated by the public's ignorance of dentistry. Because of the ADA's long-standing policy of forbidding discussions of dental quality, the public has come to believe just what we as young dental graduates once believed: One dentist is about as good as another, and one dentist's filling is about as good as another's. The public is unaware of the vast differences in the quality of service offered by different dentists, and, particularly, the public is ignorant of the disastrous consequences of substandard treatment. So the dental consumer understandably generally seeks out an economical solution to his oral problems and winds up with Dr. Poorwork, whose fees, to the unsophisticated consumer, seem to be much lower.

The young dentist soon becomes aware of this. If he is having difficulty getting patients because he is "too expensive," he might take the easy way out and become a Poorwork. And if this recent graduate is burdened with debt, he may have no choice but to join the deceitfully named swindle on the public called "managed care" (much more on this later).

Of course the economic tribulations of the Poorworks do not excuse them for the damage they do to their patients, but any attempt at reform must take their plight into account.

ENTER DR. QUACK

In the past fifteen years, one development in dentistry is at least as disturbing as Dr. Poorwork. This is the emergence of Dr. Quack.

Quackery, one of the ugliest and most noxious of human sins, has always been lucrative and requires no skill other than the ability to look your fellow human in the eye, lie to him, and take his money. This has made it attractive to many Poorworks who see it as a way out of economic hardship. We know quite a few Poorworks who have taken this road in the hope of financial salvation. Nearly every dental quack we know is a Poorwork; it seems that very few Goodworks are stooping to quackery. It may be that some Poorworks feel that incompetence in dentistry qualifies them to practice dubious medicine. (Quackery by dentists is not limited to dental concerns but also includes medical concerns well outside the boundaries of dentistry. These dental quacks are practicing medicine without a license.) Subsequent chapters probe deeply into the scams being perpetrated by dental quacks.

DR. FRAUD'S INSURANCE SCAMS

Many insurance reimbursement plans are easy to cheat, and Dr. Fraud is an expert at getting money out of these plans. He does this by reporting work that was not done, by using bait and switch and other schemes and ploys that we discuss in some detail in the chapter on managed care. What is amazing is that insurance companies make it easy for dentists to cheat. Indeed, there are even courses given to teach dentists and their office staffs how to get the maximum allowable reimbursement and also how to "pad" the bill.

Dr. Fraud siphons needed resources out of the reimbursement plans, making it more difficult for legitimate claims to be paid. To counter Dr. Fraud, the managed care administrators are forced to cut covered services and to increase co-payments and premiums.

2. The Development of Traditions and Ethics

✳

"THE POORER THE SERVICE, THE GREATER THE REWARD"

Over the years, the traditions of practice and the ethical behavior of dentists have evolved through the competitive economic environment and have been regulated and overseen by organized dentistry. One result is the published "principles of ethics," which is supposed to guide dentists' conduct. For years the ADA's "principles of ethics" set the style for dental ethics, and a dreadful style it was. One might expect a published ethical code to define proper behavior of dentists toward the public, but not this ethical code, which merely specified behavior of one dentist toward another in a manner reminiscent of "honor among thieves."

For example, dentists were not permitted to tell on one another. One dentist was not allowed to state or even gently intimate that the services of another dentist were inferior, however horrible the other dentist's work was. This led to considerable embarrassment and distress for Dr. Goodwork as he tried to explain to a patient why the tooth that Dr. Poorwork filled a year ago now needed the heavy expense of treatment with root canal and a post and crown, without citing the real reason, Poorwork's incompetence.

We recall the advice given one of us as a young dentist by an old-timer: "Sometimes you have to do what is best for yourself instead of what is best for the patient." This jibed with what an instructor in dental school said when asked why he was recommending and teaching us an expensive treatment for a situation in which a much simpler and cheaper treatment would have been at least as good: "We are not altruists," was his unforgettable reply. This open willingness to defraud a patient for your own profit was not addressed in the published ethical code, but any attempt to put the blame where it belonged for a patient's sorry condition was strictly forbidden. This helped create the atmosphere that enabled Dr. Poorwork to flourish.

Historically the healer was a person who had knowledge, abilities, and powers that set him apart from the others. To enter the fraternity of healers required privileged selection and periods of training and formal initiation, with the initiate always being sworn to secrecy. Care was taken to maintain the mystery and the distance between healer and patient. To this end a new nomenclature was developed and stringent requirements were established for the behavior of patients. Elaborate rationalizations were prepared to explain away the failure of the healer's methods. It was said, for example, that the healer never failed; instead, an evil spirit borne by the patient was at fault. Any challenge to the supremacy of the healers was countered by mumbo jumbo coupled with threats of supernatural retaliation. Such tactics were almost invariably effective and are echoed today by the use of arcane language, the reluctance of doctors to testify against one another, and the secrecy of HMO-doctor contracts.

From such beginnings today's healing arts have sprung, and a modern observer might well say that they haven't sprung very far. Today's Poorworks and Quacks commonly use these tactics to rationalize away their failures. It is the patient, never the doctor, who is at fault. "If you had only come to me early enough," or "If you had followed my directions more carefully," are typical responses to those less-timid patients who ask why their treatments were such failures. Even the legitimate professional societies still have many trappings of the secret society; they have made it difficult for the public to acquire any substantive knowledge of the inner workings of the profession. The ADA, for example, has in the past imposed complete censorship on the public writings and utterances of its members. The rationale has been that laypeople do not have the background to interpret professional information. In the hands of the public, a little knowledge is a dangerous thing, and any hard facts may be misconstrued. So it is much better to keep people ignorant of these sensitive matters. As for the patients, they can rely on the benevolent condescension of us doctors; everything will be all right as long as nobody asks any questions.

And so prescriptions are still written in Latin, usually illegible to the patient (and sometimes to the pharmacist), and doctors say "hemorrhage" instead of "bleeding" and "sequellae" instead of "consequences." Patients have been trained to suffer the rudest treatment without complaint. A patient with an appointment may wait hours until seen by the doctor. Before launching a complex treatment, the doctor often requires the patient to sign a release; he is never to be at fault, no matter what the result.

Curiously, the doctor cannot even be prosecuted for *intentional* malpractice but only for inadvertent or accidental malpractice (more on this later). The doctor is often too busy to answer questions truthfully, perhaps feeling that he would be wasting time since the patient would not understand the answer anyway. For example, a patient who asks why a filling cost $150 might be told that there actually were three fillings in the tooth. The true answer is that there was only one filling, but it was large, deep, and covered three surfaces of the tooth. But this answer might lead the patient to ask, "All that money for just one filling?" Further explanation would require the patient to try to understand the business aspect of the profession, reducing the mystery gap between doctor and patient.

The code of ethics of the dental profession seems to be a modern outgrowth of the doctor's ancient desire to keep his secrets from the public. This is achieved by never permitting the public to have access to information that might cause some unpleasant questions to be asked. Take, for example, a simple truth: A person who gives his mouth good care should rarely or never lose important teeth except, perhaps, in old age. This, in the light of modern achievements, is agreed on by good dentists everywhere. But the ADA does not want the public to know this established fact, because patients who take care of their teeth but lose them anyway might begin to question the quality of the work done by their dentists. So an elemental truth—that people should not lose teeth—is suppressed. And it is suppressed effectively: Patients who have had years of Poorwork treatment often remark that they are fifty or sixty years old and still have quite a few teeth left, and isn't that wonderful!

The traditional ethics of dentistry lead to some Alice in Wonderland results. Dr. Goodwork competently makes a routine single-surface filling in a tooth and charges his fee for it; Dr. Poorwork/Fraud might make three small pits in a similar tooth and charge three times as much for three fillings. Poorwork knows that he did an inferior job, that the tooth is odds-on to give future trouble, but he made more money in less time. One might think that such behavior is clearly unethical. Wrong! According to dental ethical traditions, as long as the immoral dentist maintains that his treatment was *in his judgment* correct, his conduct is beyond reproach. This contributes to a system of incentives that rewards haste and resultant low quality: "The poorer the service, the greater the reward!"

Now consider Dr. Goodwork, who spends more time properly restoring the tooth for one third Poorwork's fee. If he says, truthfully, that Poorwork's three-pit filling in another tooth is faulty and must be redone before trouble starts, then, according to the dental ethical tradition, he, Goodwork, is the one who is unethical! Such are the results of the traditional "ethics" of dentistry. The only one allowed to make a moral judgment on the treatment of a patient is the dentist performing the treatment. It is easy to imagine the results of such a code, and a critical examination of American dentistry today shows these results clearly.

Dr. Schissel's 1970 book *Dentistry and Its Victims* contained strong criticism of the dental ethical code of its day. The ADA responded by proposing revisions in the code. The new code does indeed refer pointedly to the dentist's responsibility to the patient and to provide quality care ("within the bounds of the clinical circumstances"). And it does reverse the previous position on judging a colleague's work, mandating that poor and immoral dentistry be reported "to the appropriate reviewing agency." *But not to the patient.* It also allows a dentist to provide expert testimony "when that testimony is essential to a just and fair disposition of a judicial or administrative action."

Shortly after the rules were revised, we reported the flagrantly immoral and incompetent behavior of a colleague to "the appropriate reviewing agency," the local ADA chapter. This kangaroo court refused either to look at the patient involved or even hear what we had to say. And we have had enough similar experiences since to conclude that the new section of the code of ethics requiring us to report "poor and immoral dentistry" is so much blather. And we are still required to engage in the cover-up of Dr. Poorwork's work to the patient.

In a letter to a dental trade magazine that had published one of our articles, the dentist-writer complained that we should not be policemen to our colleagues but instead should allow the law to weed out malpractice and fraud. Our response was that we would prefer to be judged by the court of science rather than the court of law. We would prefer to have our methods and actions judged by dentists and scientists who understand the subject than by scientifically unschooled judges and juries who are bedazzled by charismatic lawyers who are bound not to seek the truth but to serve the interests of their clients.

Dentists are now allowed to provide "expert testimony." The whole area of expert testimony is suspect. There are no scientific standards in a court of law: For money, one can find so-called experts to testify to anything you want, however scientifically absurd. Peter Huber's book *Galileo's Revenge* shows how fraudulent expert testimony, combined with what he calls "junk science," has made a travesty of justice and has cost the public millions. We recall a surgeon who was notoriously incompetent and immoral. Physicians are ordinarily loath to take action against a colleague, but this surgeon was so bad that a concerted effort was made to get rid of him, and they finally got him off the hospital staff. When we asked what happened to this surgeon, we found out that he was in another state, giving expert testimony!

Most people think that the law protects them from incompetence, fraud, and quackery. The opposite is true: The law, generally under the guise of personal freedom, actually protects the Poorworks and quacks. Malpractice actions provide an example: Remarkably enough, *intentional* dental malpractice (which Poorwork performs daily, such as leaving decay under a filling) is almost impossible to establish legally. "Malpractice" is defined as not conforming to the standards of care in the community, and in the common enough case of a community mostly of Poorworks it's virtually impossible to commit legal malpractice, however awful and negligent the treatment is. Dr. Poorwork can always say that what he did was, "in his judgment," the right thing, and, more important legally, what other dentists would do in that situation.

While it is extremely difficult to punish *intentional* malpractice, *unintentional* malpractice is actionable and fairly easy to establish legally. If a dentist, accidentally and inadvertently, drops a broken drill bit down the patient's throat, or cuts the tongue with a drill, the lawyers will pounce. As the law works, the dentist who intentionally damages a patient for profit is safe; the dentist who, while trying to serve the patient well, has an accident, is liable.

On occasion we have seen work so shamefully fraudulent and incompetent, causing damage to the patient so great and so inexcusable, that we have offered to testify at no cost if the patient decided to sue. But no patient has *ever* taken us up on it; truly victimized patients seem to be reluctant to sue their culpable dentist. Perhaps they feel foolish for having accepted and paid for such inferior care, or perhaps Poorwork was "such a nice guy," or perhaps they simply want to get the incident behind them. Whatever the reason, we have observed that patients who have genuinely been damaged are usually reluctant to sue. On the other hand, in the case of almost every patient who has come to us asking for our help in suing the previous dentist, we felt that the previous dentist had done nothing wrong. The patient's complaint was due to lack of communication with the dentist and/or unrealistic expectations of the dental procedure. Often it's something like, "I had only four teeth left, but I expected that after the treatment I would be able to chew again like I could when I was sixteen!"

Quacks actually *use* the law to promote their fraudulent activities. A jury, scientifically naive, usually gives more credence to an impressive-sounding quack than to a less charismatic scientist with more legitimate credentials. The quack always prefers to test his methods in the court of law, where his chances are excellent, rather than in the court of science, where he has no chance at all. In scientific medicine, one is *guilty until proved innocent:* A treatment is not considered appropriate for use until *after* it is proved safe and effective. In the court of science, the quack, who never can prove his methods to be safe and effective (because they aren't) always loses. But in law, he is innocent until proved guilty. The quack much prefers this approach. He likes to enter the courtroom as an innocent doctor and can usually get a few bamboozled patients, a fraudulent "expert," and his Aunt Matilda to testify that he is a fine person and that his snake oil treatment cured many a horrid case of housemaid's knee.

When a real scientist is criticized, he goes into the library and the laboratory to provide research to prove his assertions. When the quack is criticized, he finds a crooked lawyer and sues. Some years ago Dr. Dodes was scheduled to lecture to a lay audience on nutrition fraud. Before the lecture he got a call from a lawyer representing a notorious radio nutrition quack, who threatened that if Dodes even mentioned this quack in his lecture he would be sued! This type of threat stifles the free exchange of information, for while Dr. Dodes would almost certainly have eventually won the case, he would have been forced to spend enormous amounts of time and money defending himself. The radio quack, making millions of dollars, can well afford the money and loves the publicity. Even if he loses, he can claim that organized medicine and dentistry are "out to get" him. The major loser is the public, which is prevented from getting accurate and complete information on which to make critically important choices concerning their health.

And clever attorneys can make mincemeat out of a dentist's testimony. A periodontist we know once testified for a patient. Her dentist, over the years, had neglected to scale her teeth and remove tartar, and now, as a result, she was suffering periodontal disease and tooth loss.

"What studies can you cite to back your contention that tartar causes periodontal disease?" thundered the defense attorney at our colleague.

"All dental experts know and teach that tartar is an important part of the causes—"

"Perhaps you didn't hear my question," interrupted the lawyer. "Show me those studies!"

"I don't know of any such exact studies, but . . ."

"What!" howled the attorney. "You don't know! And you're supposed to be an expert!"

And the culpable Dr. Poorwork was acquitted. Of course we know that tartar must be removed if periodontal disease is to be treated successfully. But we do not perform such experiments on humans, so there are no such studies. However, a jury, not knowledgeable in dental matters, doesn't understand this. There are also no studies that scientifically demonstrate that a human being will perish if denied food and drink, and some of these lawyers could probably hoodwink a jury on that point.

If the public cannot count on fair treatment from the courts or from organized dentistry, what can a victimized patient do? Perhaps at this time the best recourse for a patient is to learn as much as possible about dentistry, particularly the differences in the way

Dr. Goodwork operates, contrasted with the methods of Dr. Poorwork, Dr. Fraud, and Dr. Quack.

For the long range, it is our hope that a truly informed public will demand changes in the traditions of practice, changes that will upgrade the performance of all dentists. Our suggestions for such changes are found throughout this book.

ORGANIZED DENTISTRY

In the United States the primary component of organized dentistry is the American Dental Association (ADA), with its national, state, and local subdivisions. There are also organizations of specialists, of quasi-specialists, of dentists interested in a particular area of study or practice, and of dentists banding together in small study groups. There is a large and influential group called the Academy of General Dentistry (AGD), which gives "credits" for attending courses, leading to awards and "honors" for accumulated credits. (These honors are meaningless, but we suppose they look good framed and hung on office walls.) There are other organizations of dentists banding together for common purpose, professional or social. There are even quite a few dental organizations set up to promote the quackery of their members! (Much more about this later.) But when we talk about organized dentistry, generally speaking, we are talking about the American Dental Association.

The ADA has, over the years, provided some truly valuable services for dentists and even, in some cases, for the public. It publishes the most prestigious peer-reviewed dental journal, the *Journal of the American Dental Association (JADA)*. Group insurance policies are available through the ADA. It has an extensive dental library with invaluable research facilities and services; we often have used these services. And the ADA has often lobbied for the public's good; for example, it has been a strong advocate of scientific fluoridation, despite the fact that fluoridation cuts down the need for dental services.

But lately too many sins of commission and omission have been having a terrible effect on dental practice. Many recent ADA policies have been actively detrimental, while in other cases the ADA's failure to act has been disastrous. We feel that the ruinous direction in which the economic climate of dentistry is heading is largely the fault of the dreadful leadership recently provided by the ADA. And it is this economic climate that is encouraging and in many cases actually *forcing* good dentists to become Poorworks.

The ADA is currently beset with many internal problems and is losing prestige. Many young dentists are not joining the organization, and the Academy of General Dentistry, a popular organization aimed at the general dentist, has changed its long-standing policy and no longer requires members also to belong to the ADA. The ADA is receiving criticism on many fronts, including the generous compensation of its officers. The president of the ADA makes, in total, more than $300,000, and the president-elect $195,000; few among the general membership are aware of this.

Some local dental organizations find more ingenious ways to squander the dues of their members. Not only do they sponsor courses in outright quackery but they also hire expensive show-biz types for "scientific" programs. In the last few years, the alleged scientific program of the Greater Long Island Dental Meeting included, besides courses in quackery, lectures by such important dental experts as Ed Koch and Maury Povitch, who were paid reputed fees of $10,000 and $15,000 respectively.

One high-ranking employee has been convicted of embezzlement. A particularly shameful chapter in ADA history involves its program of evaluating claims made by manufacturers of dental devices and materials. When the ADA gives "provisional acceptance" of a device it doesn't mean that the device was tested and approved; it simply means that the device was apparently safe but that there was insufficient evidence that it was effective for the purposes the manufacturer claimed. Of course all the so-called research is supplied by the manufacturer. The problem to the consumer relying on the integrity of the ADA seals is that the seal meaning "acceptable" looks almost exactly like the "provisional acceptance" seal, which means "not exactly."

Years ago the ADA gave provisional acceptance and accepted for advertising certain electronic devices claimed to diagnose and treat "TMJ" (see Chapter 20). Many dentists were skeptical of these claims, and after pressure from these dentists the ADA finally convened a panel of distinguished dental scientists to evaluate these contraptions. This panel studied the devices at length and prepared a peer-reviewed scientific paper for publication in the *JADA*. The panel's conclusion was exactly what we had suspected: The tested devices were not reliable for diagnosis or treatment. The ADA journal was about to publish this study but the manufacturer of the devices, reasonably concluding that publication of a study showing the product to be useless would hurt business, objected. There was talk of a threatened lawsuit, and, amazingly, the ADA backed down and didn't publish the scientific study. The authors of the study, outraged, took the paper to the *Journal of Prosthetic Dentistry*, which published it in its entirety. The *Journal of Prosthetic Dentistry* is a respected peer-reviewed journal, but without the wide circulation and influence (and susceptibility to influence?) of the *JADA*. If a threatened lawsuit can stop the publication of a legitimate scientific study, there is something wrong with the system.

The ADA has been slow to respond to complaints about "continuing education" of dentists. The ethical code mentions the obligation for dentists to keep "their knowledge and skill current." The way to keep current, of course, is to take postgraduate courses describing and evaluating new research and new techniques. The ADA has set up a system of awarding credit for taking these postgraduate courses, the idea being that Dr. Poorwork might be made to prove he is keeping up to date by accumulating these credits. In many states dentists are required to take a specific number of hours of continuing education in order to renew their dental license. (This will probably be true in every state within a few years.) Sadly, many of the courses that are given for credit are on nondental topics (how to pick stocks), or given by people without the proper expertise. And how about unscientific courses given to dentists that actually advocate quackery?

The New Age intellectual climate is replacing skepticism with credulity, and dentists are no exception. On the dental postgraduate level, courses on unproven and disproven topics are common. In the recent past we have attended lectures that *falsely* stated that silver fillings are poisonous and that TMJ (jaw joint) problems can be diagnosed by measuring the length of the legs. One particularly noxious lecture, by a chiropractor, condemned modern medications and techniques and recommended methods that were developed by the ancients. Because of the prevalence of such nonsense being taught to dentists in the guise of "continuing education," the ADA has been petitioned to ensure that courses given for ADA credit indeed have a sound scientific basis, and the ADA has responded by initiating the Continuing Education Recognition Program (CERP), which is supposed to certify a course for scientific content. The ADA claimed that this committee would ensure that dentists receive scientifically valid courses, given by legitimate and appropriate lecturers. CERP's method is to accredit the *sponsor* of the lecture, who in turn is supposed to meet certain stringent criteria. But, unhappily, here again the ADA has opted for window dressing over substance.

We soon found out that CERP certification means absolutely nothing. We wrote to CERP complaining that a recognized CERP organization, New York's First District Dental Society, was giving a course on homeopathy. If you go to the section on quackery in this book and read about homeopathy, you'll find that it has zero scientific standing and violates major laws of chemistry and physics. In addition, the dentists who were teaching this course were admitted practitioners and promoters of homeopathy, not objective evaluators. Rather than taking a stand and disciplining a group of dentists who violated CERP's own rules, return correspondence from CERP told us that our "complaint did not demonstrate substantial noncompliance with ADA CERP standards." We cringe in horror at what one would have to do in order to demonstrate *substantial* noncompliance!

We believe that if CERP won't take a position against the promotion of a fraud such as homeopathy, then any other topic will certainly be accepted. Thus there is no program to ensure that dentists don't become misled by sincere quacks or outright charlatans. And, again, the consumer is the loser.

On June 12, 1996, Governor Pataki of New York signed into law a bill promoted by the Dental Society of the State of New York (DSSNY) requiring dentists to take a certain number of continuing education courses yearly. One DSSNY spokesman said the bill "sends a message . . . that DSSNY stands for quality assurance." Another spokesman said this shows "we are serious about policing our own profession."

What nonsense! We fail to see how courses in quackery promote "quality assurance." Nor can we see how a profession can be "serious about policing" its members when it permits incompetents, quacks, and frauds to practice with impunity.

SOME GOOD NEWS, SOME BAD NEWS

Recently the ADA at long last responded to complaints about Dr. Poorwork by publishing lists of "practice parameters." Medicine has had such parameters for many years. They are intended to set the minimum limits of what a dentist must do when examining, treating, or referring a patient. The ADA cautiously notes that these parameters are for dentists' "information and *voluntary* use" (emphasis ours), but at least this is a step, however faltering, in the right direction of telling Dr. Poorwork what he should be doing.

Much of these published "parameters" are nebulous generalities about how a dentist should do the best he can and, in general, be nice and sympathetic to the patient. But buried within the blather we found two items of more than passing interest: When making a filling, "all clinically apparent caries [decay] should be removed before the restoration is placed," and when treating the gums, "clinically apparent plaque, calculus . . . should be removed." Now, leaving decay under fillings and not removing tartar are probably the two greatest sins committed by Poorwork, and now we have, finally, a clear statement by organized dentistry that Poorwork must not do this. Of course, the ADA is careful to state prominently that these parameters are not legally binding. But they do, finally, represent the first "official" message criticizing some of Poorwork's methods.

It might be mentioned here that the recent "principles of ethics" specifically condemns as unethical the popular quackery of removing silver fillings for reasons of health. The ADA has been very quiet about these pronouncements; we would like to see them widely publicized, as the first steps by the ADA to educate the public about bad dentistry. The bad news is the lack of outspoken publicity; the good news is that these statements have been made at all.

3. A Sick Profession

*

THE PLIGHT OF THE YOUNG DENTIST

I would never, never advise any young person to become a dentist today" was the upsetting reply we got when we asked a dentist if his son was going into the profession. This reflects the current sentiment of many dentists and is a profound change. In the past it was extremely common for the children of dentists to follow in their parents' footsteps. The child could expect to move into and eventually take over an active practice, without having to start up a new practice, finance a new office, and look for patients. But things have changed, and, sad to say, dentistry is no longer an attractive vocational option.

There was a time when a young dentist, just graduated, was able to go directly into private practice. Some were able to join or take over an established office, but even for those starting on their own the path was relatively easy. He rented an office, bought some furniture, got some dental equipment, hung out a shingle, and waited for patients to show up. Initial financial outlay was minimal; in those days the dentist could work alone, without an assistant at the chair or a secretary-receptionist. Equipment could be bought from the manufacturer on credit; dental manufacturers assumed, usually rightly, that the young dentist was not burdened with debt and was an excellent credit risk. The dentist could do his own bookkeeping, not complicated by insurance forms, OSHA regulations, or employee pension and medical plans. So, all alone, faced with minimal continuing expense, the dentist could sit and wait for people to come and for a practice to develop. Moreover, the dentist had control over the type of dentistry he practiced. If he chose to practice meticulous, high-quality dentistry, he could allot enough time per patient to achieve this goal. This often meant a willingness to accept a small income at first while taking the time necessary to build a reputation and to cultivate the type of patient who desires the best of care.

Today things are much different. Nowadays it is virtually impossible for a young dentist to establish such a private practice of high quality. Again, it is the economic factor that intrudes. It simply is too expensive for a recent dental graduate, unless he is a millionaire, to open a private practice. First there is the cost of undergraduate and dental school education, proportionately much higher than when we were students. The young dentist today can easily be a quarter million dollars in debt. On top of that he is faced with the expense of setting up a new office, including dental equipment and two operating rooms full of equipment. Modern equipment is designed for the dentist to be assisted by a trained chairside assistant, so a full-time assistant must be hired and trained, as well as a receptionist-secretary-bookkeeper. Modern complexities with taxes, pension and medical plans, and proliferating government regulations require the services of a professional accountant at least every few months. So, by the time this young dentist completes schooling and sets up and capitalizes the new practice, he is likely to be half a million dollars in debt. But at the start there are no patients, except for Cousin Willie and Aunt Ella, who aren't paying anyway, so at first there is no income, no way to make payment on the debts, and perhaps no way even to eat.

And there is no decent way to deal with competition. In the American free-enterprise system it is traditional to meet competition in a variety of ethical ways. One can offer a better product and/or a lower price. A new dentist can present a more caring and more pleasing personality, and can offer lower prices. But the guidelines and ethics of dentistry do not allow the new dentist to offer a better service to the public. He is not permitted to advertise or even claim in conversation that his work is superior to that of Dr. Poorwork, and this puts him at a terrible competitive disadvantage. He cannot say, "My prices are higher than my competitors because I spend more time and produce work of better quality." All he can advertise is, "Come to me and enjoy my higher prices."

All in all, it is a numbing prospect, and is the reason why only a small fraction of young dentists are able to open their own practices. The great majority of new graduates try to find jobs with existing practices. Some are lucky and obtain a position with an existing practice where high-quality dentistry is practiced. These young dentists will be able slowly to hone their skills and, with experience, gradually pick up competence and efficiency. But most recent graduates have no control over the type of dentistry they will practice. They have to subordinate their goals to the requirements of their employers, who are invariably interested in today's bottom line, not tomorrow's excellence. As an example, the licensing examinations in dentistry usually require the student to do, among other things, a routine filling on a patient. The student is allowed three hours for this routine, uncomplicated filling, and he uses the full time to execute a properly sound job. But the very next filling of this type that he does has to be accomplished not in three hours but in a few minutes! Because if he took more time, the Affordable Managed Care Family Dental Clinic, for which he is now working, would not make a profit. It is obvious that this filling cannot be properly done in such a short time by the inexperienced dentist, so economic pressures act to depress the quality of treatment, and a young dentist, faced with these pressures, cultivates sloppy treatment habits and may never develop and perfect the skills needed to efficiently perform quality dentistry. And so another Poorwork is born.

(We should mention here that an experienced dentist does not need three hours to accomplish that filling. Skill and experience could sharply reduce the necessary time for such a job, but never to a few minutes.)

A PROFESSION IN TROUBLE

Dental diseases are the most common ailments in the United States, accounting for more than $37 billion in dental bills last year. But dentistry is a profession in economic trouble, and this can spell serious difficulties for the patient as well as the dentist. Some of the things troubling dentists include: an oversupply of dentists and increased competition from advertising offices, the proliferation of third-party plans, higher costs for getting an education and opening a practice, less dental disease among the population (because of fluoridation and better oral hygiene) and the resultant lower demand for traditional dental service, diminished regard for the methods of science (on the part of dentists as well as laymen), and the refusal or inability of organized dentistry to develop strong practice guidelines and controls.

ECONOMICS: NEED, SUPPLY, AND DEMAND

Because of the ubiquitous nature of dental disease, the supply of dentists has never been enough to meet the country's dental *need.* But if we instead consider *demand,* there currently seems to be an oversupply of dentists. Dental disease is not life threatening and, rightly or wrongly, is associated in the popular mind with pain, so the demand for dental services has always been much less than the need. And economic factors operate with demand, not need. A half dozen dental schools have closed in the last few years, and many others have reduced their number of students. While this will, in time, tend to balance out supply and demand, it offers no help for the near future.

There is little doubt that fluoridation of community water supplies, which has dramatically decreased dental disease in this country, has played the major role in lessening both dental need and dental demand. Rampant decay in children's teeth is rarely seen today; a few decades ago it was quite common. The increased awareness of effective oral hygiene has further reduced disease. So today we have more dentists to treat less disease, and many dentists, hurting economically, are looking for ways to augment their income. The response of many dentists to these problems has been questionable promotional and "marketing" activities, and in too many cases dentists are also resorting to that ancient but ever effective moneymaker, quackery.

But a great many dentists are responding to the financial squeeze by signing up with managed care plans. Many dentists, feeling today's economic squeeze, are rushing to join these panels lest they be left out. These plans recruit patients by focusing on economics while disregarding quality; the only thing they promise prospective plan members is lower cost. The organization of these panels along economic lines poses a serious threat to the ability of a dentist to deliver to patients sound and appropriate treatment. (See Chapter 21.)

These plans are, at least on the surface, attractive to most patients. What could be more attractive than this typical pitch: "Tired of paying high fees to your dentist? Join our plan, get free exams, cleanings, X rays, and more, and pay up to 50 percent less in the unlikely event that you need work not included in the plan." Concealed in this pitch is the bait-and-switch fraud and the fact that these plans generally deliver dental treatment of the lowest common denominator. Nevertheless, this reasoning is proving persuasive to a great many people, and many established dentists, Goodworks and Poorworks both, have been losing patients to these plans. The newly graduated dentists trying to establish a practice have found the pool of available new patients greatly diminished by the popularity of these plans. Slowly but progressively, these plans are beginning to control the supply of patients.

And to control the supply of patients is to control the economic behavior of the doctors. It is easy to see that, in the future, the bottom-line-oriented insurance plan that controls the patients of a dentist's practice will be able to say to that dentist something like this: "We think you're making too much money, so we're cutting your fees in half." The dentist will be helpless to resist. With the third party controlling the supply of patients, the doctor will either have to bend to the demands of the third party or starve.

(As this is being written, Aetna Insurance is trying to get its plan-member physicians to accept a "capitation" reimbursement plan that not only will sharply reduce doctors' incomes but also severely cut down on the quality of care they are able to provide. Aetna may control enough patients to accomplish this.)

If a managed care plan that controls most of the patient supply of a particular dentist suddenly decides to reduce the dentist's fees, the dentist has two choices: lose most of his patients, or accept the lower fees. If he accepts the lower fees, to maintain his income he will have to see many more patients, "increase production" in the jargon of practice management. This means that he will have to speed up his work—and speed is the death of good dentistry. The bottom line for this dentist will therefore be either to lose most of his patients and starve or become a Poorwork! Not a pleasant predicament for an ethical dentist, but what choices does he have? Particularly shameful is the fact that his own professional organization, the American Dental Association, has no help or remedy for him. The ADA will not lift a finger to save Dr. Goodwork if it means exposing Dr. Poorwork. And so, faced with these problems, the sick profession gets sicker, and in the near future it may become impossible for a patient to receive competent dental care unless he can find the rare professional who resists joining the plans and is able to still make a living. It may well be that good dentistry will soon become a rare and very expensive commodity.

THE VALUE OF GOOD DENTISTRY

The question comes up whether truly good dentistry is worth all the extra time it takes, or are we dealing with diminishing returns. The answer lies in an examination of the long-range results of dental practice. The results of a high-quality local practice started in 1924 offer some characteristic insight. With very few exceptions, long-standing patients of this practice have kept their teeth; an extraction is a very rare event for these patients, and, except for wisdom teeth, most of them have never experienced an extraction. And dental restorations (fillings, bridges, etc.) in this practice enjoy substantial longevity. *Every good-quality dental practice can tell the same story.* Dr. Poorwork, on the other hand, has very few successes to boast about. Most of his patients suffer through repeated dental procedures (all of them done hastily), continuing discomfort and pain, and repeated expense, and finally wind up with full or partial dentures. Good dentistry is well worth the extra time and effort, and usually turns out to be more economical over the long run, since carefully done dental procedures show excellent longevity and rarely fail or have to be done over. Good dentistry not only saves money but also preserves dental health.

It would be nice to be rid of Dr. Poorwork altogether, but the American Dental Association has never been willing to do what is required. Many good dentists are complaining that they are losing patients to managed care schemes, which purport to be much cheaper. Time will tell if economic forces compel Dr. Goodwork to adopt hasty methods. Gresham's Law of economics describes how bad money drives out good money; similarly, under the economic conditions imposed by managed care (the poorer the service, the greater the reward), bad dentistry is driving out good dentistry. And so the sick profession gets sicker. Its primary disease is not only Dr. Poorwork but also the organizational system that permits Poorwork to exist and even thrive. Worse yet, this system is evolving into a blueprint to make it difficult for Dr. Goodwork to survive without turning himself into Dr. Poorwork.

One might think that the ADA, a mighty professional organization representing 130,000 American dentists, would give some time and thought to the plight of dentists who wish to continue to produce a quality service but are being forced by economic factors to debase the way they treat their patients. But, alas, the ADA also represents Dr. Poorwork and hasn't the guts to do what is necessary to protect the profession.

The trend in our population's oral health has been positive. A 1971 survey showed that in the age category fifty-five to sixty-four the typical citizen had lost more than half his teeth. A 1985 survey showed the same citizen with 37 percent of the teeth missing. We expect that this positive trend is continuing, considering the effectiveness of fluoridation and improved dental techniques. But, as the sick profession gets sicker, and high-quality dental services become more scarce, will this trend reverse?

4. Why Good Dentists Turn Bad

*

Why do good dentists turn bad? In a word, money. The economic climate in dentistry makes it difficult—and in some cases impossible—to practice first-class dentistry and still make a living. On the other hand, in the same kind of economic atmosphere Dr. Poorwork can prosper. Compounding this problem is organized dentistry's policy to prevent the public's access to essential information about dentistry. The public, thinking that Poorwork's treatment is just as good as Goodwork's, understandably goes for the cheaper treatment. In the past, many dentists resisted the financial incentives to cheapen their quality and become Poorworks, but many didn't. The situation today is considerably worse!

Too many patients have found dentistry to be merely a series of pain-relieving treatments while, over the years, they gradually lose their teeth. The dentist relieved pain and put in new teeth to replace the teeth extracted. After all, isn't it natural to lose teeth as you grow older? Largely because of organized dentistry's hush-hush policy, these people have never learned that they should not have lost their teeth, and that lost teeth almost always means personal neglect and/or poor dentistry.

With this in mind, allow us to develop a scenario illustrating the risks of trying to do the best dentistry. Suppose a dentist opens a practice in a typical, mixed white-collar and working-class neighborhood. Young Dr. Goodwork wants his new neighbors to become his patients. Time-honored economic practice dictates that to attract customers Goodwork must generate demand, and demand characteristically is for dentistry that is quick, cheap, and painless (another way of describing Dr. Poorwork's methods). Our new dentist realizes that if he lets the word out that he will meet this demand, he may soon be blessed with a lively low-quality practice. But he is still young and idealistic and believes that he should be able to educate his patients to welcome good work, despite the attitude of the ADA. After all, in the long run doesn't good work maintain a healthy mouth, and doesn't it involve less pain and inconvenience, and isn't it probably less costly? And so Goodwork sets about presenting his conception of good dentistry to his new patients—and immediately runs into the first risk of performing good dentistry.

THE RISK OF BEING CONSIDERED EXPENSIVE

Dr. Goodwork has a new patient willing to give the young dentist a try. The patient accepts his higher fee for a complete examination and indeed notices that Goodwork's examination is so much more thorough than was Poorwork's. But if the former dentist was indeed a Poorwork, there is a good chance that the patient will need substantial remedial and restorative work, at high cost. He may need faulty fillings replaced, abscessed teeth treated, missing teeth replaced, and neglected gum disease treated. The patient is likely to be staggered by the stated fee. After all, Dr. Poorwork, at his last exam, never said he needed anything like this much work! So, from Dr. Goodwork's first contact with people in the neighborhood, the word spreads that he is expensive, even though his fees actually represent a spectacular bargain when compared on a time-and-result basis with those of Dr. Poorwork.

THE RISK OF BEING CONSIDERED A "CON MAN"

Goodwork's efforts to justify his higher fees are frustrating. He cannot tell the patient the truth, that while he intends to provide first-class services Dr. Poorwork never did, which is why so much work is needed. Goodwork is restricted to a dispassionate presentation of the patient's existing condition, the need for correction, and the planned treatment. He can show charts, diagrams, slides, models, videos; he can discuss dental theory at length; he can claim that his treatment will save the teeth and, in the long run, even save money. But, the patient will ask, isn't this exactly what his old dentist, Dr. Poorwork, has been doing all along, and at half the cost? The "ethics" of dentistry prohibit Goodwork from giving the candid answer the question needs, and the patient walks out, reporting that the young dentist is a fast-talking con man trying to sweet-talk people into a lot of work at high fees.

THE RISK OF BEING ACCUSED OF PRESCRIBING UNNECESSARY WORK

When Dr. Goodwork prescribes loads of expensive work, while Dr. Poorwork, at his last exam six months ago never mentioned anything like this, the patient may go back to Poorwork, who may say in his opinion all that work isn't needed. Now the word spreads that Goodwork is building up business by prescribing expensive work that is not necessary. The very nature of dental disease helps Dr. Poorwork, because it often takes many years for the poor-quality rushed work that Poorwork produces to cause the problems that high-quality work could have avoided. So while the patients of Poorwork may someday learn the sad truth, enlightenment usually comes too late to save their teeth and too late to save Dr. Goodwork's reputation.

THE RISK OF BEING CONSIDERED A PAINFUL DENTIST

The fear of pain has caused many people to avoid periodic dental treatment altogether, and a reputation for inflicting pain can be fatal to a practice. Nevertheless, compared with Dr. Poorwork's superficial methods, some of Goodwork's procedures are going to produce discomfort, most often after the work is completed. The deep scalings used to treat gum conditions often leave the gums sore and tender for a day or so. Dr. Poorwork's five-minute "cleanings" and chemical "gum treatments" never hurt anybody, at least not until the teeth loosen from periodontal disease. When Goodwork fills a tooth, he drills deeply enough to remove all decay and to prepare the tooth properly for the restoration. These deep fillings can be sore for a few days and harbor sensitivity to hot and cold for much longer. Dr. Poorwork's fillings, with a minimum of drilling and, too often, with much of the decay left in, rarely hurt—until the tooth abscesses, which may not happen for years.

X-ray examination often shows Dr. Goodwork a lot of decay

that has been left under a filling made by Dr. Poorwork. Though the tooth still shows no symptoms, Goodwork knows that if he does not act at once, it will soon require at least a costly root canal treatment with possibly a post and crown, or, at worst, the tooth may be nonrestorable and have to be extracted. At this moment the tooth may be at the point where the decay is breaking through to the pulp (the inner material commonly called the "nerve"), where an influx of bacteria will cause an abscess. Dr. Goodwork begins the arduous and delicate job of removing all decay and trying to avoid a pulp involvement. This is a job, Dr. Goodwork ruefully observes, that would have been easy when the filling was first done, before the decay had spread. But Poorwork never took the time to properly clean the tooth of decay, and now Goodwork is breaking his back for close to an hour trying to save this tooth.

This situation has many possible results. Suppose Dr. Goodwork happily is able to complete the job without a pulpal involvement, and he places a well-made filling. Since he took close to an hour to complete this filling, he will have to charge considerably more than Poorwork did for his five-minute botch of the same tooth, so the patient is already likely to be resentful. Then, this tooth may be sensitive for several weeks. And there is a small possibility that the tooth may abscess anyway in response to the heavy presence of bacteria-laden decay close to the pulp. If, while removing the decay, Dr. Goodwork found that decay had gotten into the pulp, he might try a pulp-capping, a simple procedure that is often successful. But sometimes the outcome of this procedure lies in the balance for months, then failing and requiring root canal. In any case, the patient is likely to experience discomfort.

Now how does all of this sit with the new patient? Poorwork's solution to the tooth's problem would be to disregard the decay under the filling until the tooth began to show symptoms, then to announce to the patient that the tooth had "gone bad" and had to be extracted. And extractions, done with anesthetics, don't hurt. Also remember that two years ago Poorwork had easily filled this tooth in a few minutes, and it had never hurt until Goodwork got his hands on it. So the word goes out again: Goodwork means pain and trouble.

THE RISK OF BEING CONSIDERED AN INEPT AMATEUR

The average patient is not equipped to judge a dentist's ability. The patient in the previous example may well believe that Dr. Goodwork's skill is seriously wanting. He takes much longer to do his work, he sweats and strains and mutters to himself, and the patient experiences discomfort. The legendary criterion of "gentle hands" cannot be sympathetically applied by one who has been sitting in a chair, mouth open and cheeks contorted, for almost an hour. But twenty years hence a patient of Dr. Goodwork may adopt a better standard of judgment when he notices that he still has all his teeth in good condition, while his friends, loyal to Dr. Poorwork, are in discomfort, can't chew as well, and are missing many teeth. But Goodwork may not find it possible to wait a generation for people to appreciate him. And meanwhile the standard of competence continues to be Dr. Poorwork, a dentist so skillful that he fills teeth quickly and painlessly. And the word goes out: Goodwork is clumsy and incompetent.

While we have detailed some of the risks of doing good dentistry, one might ask if there are any risks in doing substandard dentistry à la Poorwork. The answer is no, not as long as the "ethics" of dentistry have conditioned people to view the loss of teeth as an inevitable part of the aging process. Just as the bad surgeon buries his incompetent work, so Dr. Poorwork extracts his. And he makes a nice living in the process.

5. Quality: The Essential but Forgotten Factor

*

There is nothing a person cannot make a little worse and sell a little cheaper, and those who go by price alone are this man's lawful prey.

—Dr. Charles H. Mayo

American dentistry has long been considered to be the world's finest. Unique among the professions, high-quality American dentistry has developed the technical means to solve virtually every dental health problem. With very few exceptions, a person practicing decent oral hygiene and receiving good dental care enjoys a lifetime of well-functioning, comfortable, and good-looking teeth. Even in old age a person should continue to be able to enjoy eating and properly nourish himself with healthy natural teeth.

But, when we look around us, we find that this is not true. Too many people reaching middle age have already lost many, or most, or all of their teeth. How does this reality accord with the rosy picture just painted? What is the fly in the ointment?

To this question there are many answers and many factors contributing to these answers, and they are all contained within the word "quality." Woven through the fabric of this book is the concept of quality, the preeminent factor that relates to everything about dentistry: dental practice, dental insurance, dental overhead, dental fees, dental home care, and, particularly, the search by the dental consumer for effective dental treatment.

To be blunt, only high-quality dentistry consistently achieves the felicitous result of long-term healthy teeth. Mediocre care is much less likely to preserve the teeth, and low-quality care is worth less than nothing because it often actually accelerates the loss of teeth.

But nobody talks about quality. In all the discussions about the future of the dental delivery system, the government plans, the various types of insurance coverage, the managed care systems both projected and existing, the idea of quality has been forgotten. Yet quality is the central, critical component of effective dental treatment; dentistry without quality is a waste of time, health, and resources. Rather than being kept concealed, quality is the first thing that should be put on the table when discussing any dental plan.

Oddly enough, quality in dentistry is not expensive. Though initially more costly, over the long haul it is probably less expensive than poor care, and it is certainly more effective. As an example, most insurance companies will pay for a new crown three or five years after a previous crown had been made on the same tooth. But a properly made and fitted crown can last indefinitely; good crowns rarely fail. Obviously, even if the insurance company had to pay twice as much for the good crown initially, the expense of remaking the cheap crown every few years is so much greater. And so it goes in every phase of dentistry: The high-quality restoration lasts and preserves the teeth; the cheap job must be re-done, and redone, finally losing the tooth and requiring another more elaborate restoration, which if also poorly done, will fail, causing more damage, with the dismal cycle persisting until many dollars later the patient has run out of teeth, while insurance premiums escalate. It is ironic to note that at any point in this chronicle the intercession of high-quality treatment could alter the sad result.

But, as we have said, the bottom-line mentality of insurance companies, politicians, and union officials is not trained to look at long-term results, only at today's balance sheet. And so the consumers, thinking they are getting a good deal, are deceived and ill served.

Many are the tributaries that contribute to the ocean of the quality problem. The underpinning of most is economics. Historically, in most communities, it has been more profitable to do hasty, bad dentistry than to practice high-quality dentistry. Today, with the torrent of third-party plans inundating the profession, in many situations it is becoming economically impossible to practice high-quality dentistry. The chances of a newly graduated dentist setting up a high-quality practice are slim to almost nonexistent. In areas where much of the population is signed up with union or managed care third-party plans, the third parties negotiate what they consider to be the most favorable (i.e., the least expensive) terms from the participating dentists. And these third-party plans, controlling the supply of patients to the dentist, come to hold a sword over the head of the dentist. Usually the fees paid to dentists by these plans would not cover the overhead of a quality practice but would allow a profit to a low-quality, high-volume, hasty practice. And too many dentists, these days, are being forced into this type of practice.

"Well," the despairing consumer might ask, "will I ever be able to find a high-quality dentist? And how can I know if the dentist I find really is good? Am I being cheated? And is it possible to set up a third-party plan that delivers high quality?" In this book we explore in depth every angle of this question and supply answers and suggestions. There are still good dentists to be found. There are ways to differentiate between Dr. Goodwork and the public nemeses Dr. Poorwork, Dr. Quack, and Dr. Fraud. And there are ways for people knowledgeable about the issues to influence legislation and demand quality programs from unions, insurers, government, and all third parties. It is our hope that this book is a comprehensive source for all the information needed by the consumer seeking effective dental care.

Quality in dentistry is the type of care that enables patients to keep their teeth and maintain a healthy, comfortable, functioning, and good-looking mouth. Quality means careful and complete examination leading to sound diagnosis and the selection of an appropriate long-term treatment plan. Quality means prevention. Quality means removal of oral disease and its causes. Quality means patient education. Quality means complete removal of decay and weakened structure from teeth prepared for restoration. Quality means restorations of proper form, function, bite, and appearance. Quality means rejection of fad or quack techniques, however profitable they are. And, particularly, quality means the careful planning and meticulous execution of dental procedures to produce these results. These are the methods taught in dental schools, and these are the methods used by good dentists everywhere. Quality also means continual upgrading of knowledge and skills by keeping abreast of current research.

LONGEVITY OF DENTAL WORK

Patients are understandably concerned about what to expect with their dental work. How long will a filling last? A fixed bridge? Is it better to get a crown than a filling? Longevity of dental work depends on how well the work was done and how well the patient cares for it. The following discussion assumes that both the dentistry and the patient's oral hygiene are high quality.

Amalgam fillings: As a general rule, the larger the filling, the less natural tooth remains to support it, and the higher the possibility that a supporting wall of the tooth will crack off and a crown needed. However, we routinely see large silver-amalgam fillings twenty-five to fifty years old and sometimes even older! A large amalgam should last a good quarter century, and smaller fillings could do even better.

Plastic composite fillings: Old-fashioned silicate cement fillings (commonly mislabeled "porcelain" fillings) used to be made for front teeth, since silver is unsightly. These fillings failed after several years, because the material tended to discolor and dissolve out in the saliva. But the last twenty-five years have seen dramatic improvements in tooth-colored composite filling materials, which in front teeth are quite color stable and appear to be able to last as long as amalgams. The use of composites for back teeth is becoming more popular, but the prognosis for those fillings is poorer than for amalgam. Composite materials are constantly being improved, but at this writing amalgam is still preferred for large back teeth fillings.

Crowns: A crown can be expected to last nearly a lifetime.

Bridgework: Carefully done fixed bridgework (missing teeth replaced by false teeth attached to crowns on neighboring teeth) has an excellent track record. Since failure of a crown involved in the bridge usually means failure of the bridge, the prognosis of a bridge is not as good as that of single crowns. Nevertheless, a fixed bridge can last twenty-five years and longer. But poorly done fixed bridgework has a high rate of early failure. In many cases the patient would be much better off without the poorly done bridge, which actually hastened his loss of teeth.

Implants: Implants are too new to estimate long-range prognosis, but there are many successful cases ten years old. The new titanium-based implants are a significant improvement over the old-style implants, which had a failure rate of close to 100 percent!

Root canal: Root-canal-treated teeth can last as long as teeth that did not require the treatment. Even the root-canal-treated tooth badly damaged by decay can be saved.

Periodontal treatment: The success of competent gum treatment depends on how serious the condition was before treatment and how virulent the disease, as well as patient cooperation with excellent oral hygiene. But it is clear that periodontal treatment saves teeth that would otherwise be lost.

THE EXTENT OF THE DAMAGE

How widespread is Dr. Poorwork? There are no reliable statistics to guide us. Some insurance programs have developed a few measurements of quality, and the results have not been flattering to dentistry, but these data have been fragmentary. The American Dental Association has been no help, and its constituent societies have actually resisted attempts to study quality. This is understandable, since Dr. Poorwork also is an ADA member, and the ADA rule prohibiting criticism of other dentists supports the fiction that all dentists maintain high standards of care. A candid conversation with a practicing dentist will provide a better understanding of the quality picture than does the ADA fiction. In Dr. Schissel's *Dentistry and Its Victims,* he provided his own personal observations: "Of patients coming for initial examination, the great majority had dental restorations that did not meet the standards of dental school or the state board licensing examinations. A high proportion of this poor work fell so far short of minimum standards as to be disgraceful. Patients with this type of care can usually look forward to frequent pain and, over the years, progressive loss of teeth."

Now, twenty-five years later, Dr. Schissel can only comment that, because of the economic climate, things are even worse.

To get a clearer concept of how quality requirements affect practice, let us consider one of the most common everyday dental procedures: a two-surface silver filling on a back tooth. Here are the major steps:

1. Complete removal of decay. Active decay left in a cavity will, over a period of time, spread, progressively eating away the tooth until it can be saved only by elaborate and costly procedures. In a matter of months or years, a tooth improperly cleaned of decay will either be lost or, if the patient is lucky, it may be saved, though with great difficulty. Yet there are many well-respected, prosperous dentists who *routinely* fail to remove decay from teeth because to do so takes too much time.

2. Removal of weakened tooth structure. This is that part of the tooth that has been weakened by loss of foundation tissue, for example, sound tooth surface with its underpinnings decayed away. Areas thus weakened should be cut away before restoring the tooth. Otherwise the weakened area is likely to chip or fracture with use. Teeth with translucent, off-color areas are often the result of failure to remove undermined *enamel.*

3. Proper extension of cavity form. This is the preparation of the tooth to receive the filling; it involves considerations of both physics and physiology. There must be a sufficient mass cut from the tooth to allow for enough bulk of filling material. Broken fillings are often a result of inadequate bulk of filling material at critical areas. From the physiological point of view, the preparation must extend to all areas of the tooth that are prone to decay in the future. This principle, known to dentists as *extension for prevention,* is one of the oldest tenets of sound dentistry. Failure to observe this principle considerably increases the chance of recurrent decay around the filling.

4. Insulation or lining. This refers to the placement of a material over the deepest and presumably most sensitive area of the prepared tooth prior to placing the filling. Lining reduces thermal and mechanical shock to the pulp. Bonded materials are effective insulators.

5. Placement of the filling. In a typical two-surface filling, a band is placed around the tooth as a mold for the plugging

of the silver amalgam. The band should be wedged against the tooth beneath the gum level to help provide for flush margins between tooth and filling. The tooth must remain completely dry and clean while being filled (moisture contaminating the amalgam during placement weakens the completed filling). The amalgam must be firmly packed against the walls and floors of the preparation, and on the margins. The excess mercury in the amalgam tends to rise to the surface. This must be removed and the filling overpacked with fresh amalgam, which must then be very well packed. Finally, the band is removed and the filling is evened to the proper size.

6. If bonding techniques are to be used (see Chapter 9), several additional steps must be done to prepare the tooth for the placement of the adhesive chemicals.

7. Marginal adaptation. This is a critical yet often-neglected task. All margins of a filling must be finished flush with the tooth. An overextended filling must be trimmed, or the filling must be redone. A bad margin can destroy the soft tissue and bone support around a tooth, catch and trap food, and lead to root decay.

8. Restoration of the tooth to proper bite, form, and function. The bite is checked and rechecked and adapted until it is perfect. The filling is shaped to conform to proper anatomical size and shape for best function. Contacts with other teeth are restored and shaped until the tooth looks like a tooth again and not a shapeless glob of silver amalgam.

Obviously a "simple" filling of a moderately decayed tooth is a complicated and time-consuming procedure. Inattention to any of these details results in a substandard filling that has much less chance of ultimate success and should not be in your mouth or anybody's mouth. Yet the Dr. Poorworks do not pay enough attention to any of the steps detailed above.

It is a pernicious fact that some dental treatments are more lucrative in respect to time spent than are others, and this can have a bearing on the diagnosis. Shall the dentist do procedure A for the patient when he can make twice the money by doing procedure B? For the dentist of integrity this is not a problem. But in our current climate of bottom-line mentality, how long can integrity persist, especially in the face of managed care plans that almost force a dentist, in order to survive, to manipulate a diagnosis in the direction of profit?

For instance, replacing teeth provides a much greater financial return per time spent than filling a tooth. Why should a dentist spend hours painstakingly filling several badly decayed teeth when managed care will pay ten times as much to extract those teeth and make a removable denture, a process that is considerably easier, requires less skill, and takes much less time? And why should Dr. Poorwork work hard to fill a tooth perfectly when he gets paid so little for it? He gets paid just as much for a quick, sloppy job. And then there will be another job to be done on that tooth in a few years, then another, then an extraction, then a bridge—all done badly, but all at a fee. How can we hope to have good dentistry when bad work is more lucrative than good, and the bad dentist so well protected by the ethics of dentistry and by the American Dental Association? This reasoning has always been irresistible to Dr. Poorwork, but these days it is becoming a matter of survival for too many dentists trapped in the managed care economy.

One more insidious point: There have been very tentative beginnings of quality discussions in the profession and among managed care providers. These mostly take the stance that judgments of quality must take into account the local factors of practice. This means, to be blunt, that the dentist shouldn't be judged by absolute quality standards but by what is "good enough" for a certain community. That means that Poorwork is not acceptable for one community but is perfectly okay for another (presumably less affluent) area.

Perhaps the ultimate of this kind of thinking is demonstrated by a case study done on an indigent young woman at a dental school many years ago. According to the report written in a dental journal, after the experiment was completed the woman's teeth were all extracted "for socio-economic reasons."

POORWORK DENTAL LABS

For many major restorative operations, the dentist relies on a dental laboratory, where technicians make crowns, inlays, and a variety of custom dental products. The dentist prepares the patient's mouth and teeth to receive the restoration, takes impressions and measurements, and sends them to the laboratory where technicians prepare what the dentist needs. The laboratory work must also be of high quality to produce meticulous and precise results. But what of Dr. Poorwork? No matter how careful a lab is, it cannot possibly provide the accurate work necessary for a proper restoration from Poorwork's sloppy tooth preparation and poor impressions. So Poorwork tends to gravitate toward poorwork laboratories, which turn out cheap, *approximate* results.

POORWORK SPECIALISTS

One of the great problems facing legitimate specialists occurs when a patient is referred from a Poorwork. Often the specialist knows that whatever treatment he provides this patient won't succeed long term; Poorwork's incompetence will sabotage the result. Some specialists actually tell the patient that his best course is to leave Dr. Poorwork and find another dentist. This can be ticklish, because if there aren't any Goodworks in the neighborhood, this dries up a major source of referrals. Some specialists bite their tongues and do the best they can under the circumstances, knowing that their results will be compromised.

There are also Poorworks among specialists, dentists who attract patients by charging less than other specialists and by doing a hasty, perfunctory, and ineffectual job. On those occasions when Dr. Poorwork refers to a specialist, he is generally careful to select a Poorwork specialist who won't give him away and will cover up his incompetence. This amounts to a collusion between the two Poorworks.

Some years ago we saw a young woman whose mouth had virtually been destroyed by a Poorwork. We told her that her gum condition was serious and before we could undertake any restorative procedures she would need treatment by a periodontist, to whom she was duly referred. But the woman's mother interceded and insisted her daughter go to her periodontist; we had no objection since we assumed that this periodontist was legitimate. Several months passed, and then the patient showed up at the office telling us that her periodontal surgery had been completed and she was ready for restorations. But one look in her mouth showed us that surgery had never been done, and the periodontal condition was worse than ever! We called the periodontist, and the following unforgettable conversation ensued, in almost these exact words.

"The patient tells us that surgery is completed and she's ready for restorations."

"That's right. You can replace the five missing teeth on the upper right by a fixed seven-unit two-abutment bridge, using the central and the second molar for abutments. On the left side you can make a four-unit bridge—"

"But" we interrupted, "even with strong abutments such a bridge is unsound, and to do fixed bridges on such periodontally involved teeth is hopeless. The work won't last a year!"

"Doctor, you can count on me. I have told the patient that while the outcome is very doubtful, this work is the only chance, however slim, to save her teeth. I have prepared her for failure. The patient is willing to go ahead. Doctor, you can count on me!"

In almost so many words, this specialist was suggesting collusion not only to defraud this patient but also to destroy any chances she had for a well-functioning mouth. The economic temptations are compelling: The seven-unit bridge based on only two supporting teeth would have been easy to make, and lucrative. In effect, he was telling us that if we sent him a patient for his brand of token treatment he would send us back a lucrative restorative case that we wouldn't have to worry about because he prepared the patient for failure. Furthermore, the patient would be pleased, because the periodontal treatment (essentially not doing anything) would be painless. This specialist, believe it or not, had a respectable standing among many local dentists (probably all of them Poorworks) and was active in the politics of the local dental society.

How can quality dentistry be found? Since professional advertising is now legal, can an advertisement point the way to a quality dentist? Probably not, because of the limitations of what can be advertised. Dr. Goodwork might like to publish an ad like this: "Is your dentist producing the best dentistry? Good dentistry requires time and effort. In my practice I take the extra time needed to produce results superior to those produced by many other dentists. Of course, that means I have to charge more, but if you come to me, in the long run you will probably save money and, more important, save your teeth."

This ad, however reasonable it seems, is not permitted by the advertising guidelines and regulations of organized dentistry. For Dr. Goodwork's advertisement to fall within the guidelines it would have to read, "Come to me and take advantage of my higher prices." Quite a practice builder, that.

Amazingly enough, there is nothing in the guidelines to stop a dentist from advertising quackery! Dentists have advertised all kinds of unscientific services. (See Chapter 20.)

The following chapters give consumers, dentists, and managed care administrators the tools to evaluate the quality of the dental treatment they are paying for.

Part II

*

For the Dental Consumer

6. The Basics

THE MOUTH: THE PRIMARY ANIMAL ORGAN

We call the mouth the primary animal organ because early animals were mouths and not much more. As evolution proceeded, organs and appendages were added to assist the mouth in its main purpose: to nourish the animal. It is interesting to note that in humans, because of its central importance, there are many more nerves per area serving the mouth than any other part of the body.

The mouth is extraordinarily complex and, needless to say, vitally important for life. It allows us to eat, taste, drink, breathe, and express ourselves. So when something goes wrong with the mouth, the whole body tends to suffer. The mouth includes the lips, the tongue, the cheeks, the teeth, and the muscles of chewing, which taken together are the complete apparatus for ingesting food. The mouth also contains salivary glands that produce a fluid (saliva) with remarkable properties, and at the back of the mouth is the valve that routes food and air into the proper internal systems. The mouth can also endure temperatures ranging from the freezing point of ice cream to the scalding heat of soup. Amazingly, the mouths of healthy people regularly play host to more than eighty varieties of microorganisms, many of which would produce serious infections in other parts of the body. We will fastidiously forbear discussing the role assigned to the mouth by the Freudians.

The tongue is a strong, active muscle, only part of which is under conscious control. It assists in the placement of food for chewing and is essential for swallowing and speaking. The tongue is so strong that if it habitually presses on one or more teeth, it can cause them to move.

The jaw muscles, which are used for chewing, are exceeded in strength only by the calf muscles of the legs. The jaw muscles, using the teeth, can chew through bones, tear the cap off a beer bottle, or even enable a circus performer to swing while held by the teeth! (We do not recommend any of these exercises.) On the inside of each cheek is a small lump that is the duct of the parotid salivary gland. In some people, a bony protrusion called a torus can grow in the midline of the palate or on both inside aspects of the lower jaw. (These lumps are normal; we mention them because often people becoming aware of their presence for the first time are afraid that these lumps are cancers. They are not.)

The most significant protective factor in the mouth is the saliva, which is produced continuously, keeping the mouth from drying out. It lubricates the food, making chewing and swallowing easier, and it begins the digestion of starches. It also contains chemicals that fight infections and can neutralize both acids and bases, thus protecting the sensitive oral tissues from damage. Saliva is an amazing disinfectant (ask your cat). A gaping wound anywhere on the body, other than in the mouth, is very likely to become infected. Yet the large hole left in the gum and bone following a tooth extraction almost always heals without problems.

The teeth are composed of hard, calcified tissues. The one third of the tooth you can see is called the crown; the rest, buried under the gums, is called the root. The crown is covered with a very hard substance called enamel, which is similar to fingernails in that it is not "alive" and contains no nerve fibers. Enamel is the hardest naturally occurring substance except for diamonds. Under the very hard enamel is the slightly less hard dentin, which is very similar to bone. Dentin does contain nerve fibers, making it painful when decay (or drilling) gets this deep. Within the dentin is a hollow space called the pulp chamber and pulp canal, which contain the pulp. The pulp is the tissue commonly known as the "nerve" because it is so very sensitive, but it actually consists of connective tissue and blood vessels in addition to nerve fibers. The dentin of the root is covered with a special hard material called cementum. Microscopic elastic fibers, called periodontal ligament fibers, go from the cementum to the jawbone and hold the tooth firmly in its socket. These fibers, the gums, and the surrounding jawbone are called the periodontal tissues. A breakdown of these tissues that support the teeth is known as periodontal disease.

The pulp has the ability to form new dentin, called secondary dentin, which it does in response to the irritation of decay or

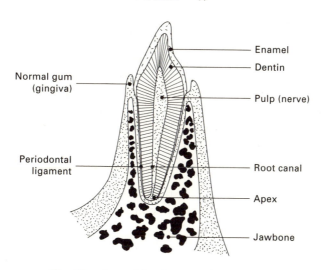

The Tooth and Its Supporting Tissues

trauma. This ability allows the tooth to set up a wall against the progress of caries (decay). This race is always won by the decay, but the defense thrown up by the pulp often gives the dentist enough time to intervene and supply a happy ending to the drama.

COMMON DENTAL PROBLEMS

Burning Mouth Syndrome

Burning mouth syndrome (BMS) is a chronic oral-facial pain syndrome that affects more than one million American adults, mostly postmenopausal females. It is characterized by a burning sensation, dry mouth, thirst, altered taste perception, changes in eating habits, irritability, depression, and a decreased desire to socialize. The most commonly affected areas are the lips, palate, and tongue. Symptoms vary widely and can go away unpredictably. Most troubling is the lack of any universally effective medication.

A number of oral and systemic disorders may contribute to the problem. Poorly fitting full dentures can lead to irritation and BMS. About 20 percent of BMS patients have measurably less saliva, a condition called *xerostomia*. The xerostomia is often due to medications, not to classic BMS.

Snoring and Sleep Apnea

Apnea is an interruption or cessation of breathing. It most often occurs during sleep. In the most common form, obstructive sleep apnea, an individual stops breathing as many as seventy times per hour. These short episodes can each last as long as thirty seconds and can deprive the person of needed oxygen and rest, leading to daytime sleepiness and altered cardiopulmonary function. Sufferers from sleep apnea not only snore heavily but are chronically drowsy. They have trouble staying awake through a movie, play, or even a TV show, and can fall asleep while driving. It is estimated that 2 to 4 percent of middle-aged adults are affected by this condition.

Most people who suffer from obstructive sleep apnea also snore, though not all people who snore have obstructive sleep apnea. Snoring is the result of vibration of the soft palate and the adjacent structures of the throat and is caused by narrowing and thickening of the upper airway tissues. Snoring can be complicated by overweight, hypertension, cardiopulmonary problems, craniofacial abnormalities, tonsillar overgrowth, genetic factors, and aging because of loss of tissue tone.

A fairly inexpensive intra-oral device that is custom fitted by a dentist has been shown to be useful for the treatment of snoring and early sleep apnea. The device opens the airway by keeping the lower jaw slightly open and forward. Most patients report substantial improvement at first, but some find the device to lose effectiveness after a period of time, ranging from months to three years, probably because of the thickening with age of the airway tissues.

Surgery has been tried with lasers and other techniques, with inconsistent results. We feel that surgery should be tried only as a last resort.

The most effective treatment by far is the use of an air pump, called a CPAP, which forces air through the nose while you sleep. The CPAP successfully deals with most cases of apnea and, as a bonus, eliminates snoring. Many CPAP patients report that they are now wide awake; they claim that they no longer fall asleep at the theater or at the wheel and have stopped snoring. A CPAP should be prescribed and fitted only after a careful evaluation is done by a physician specializing in sleep disorders.

Tobacco-Related Diseases

Tobacco has special meaning to dentists because many patients not only smoke but also chew tobacco. Chewing tobacco, also known as smokeless tobacco (ST), has been strongly associated with nicotine addiction and an increased risk of developing oral cancer. More than five million Americans are estimated to use ST, resulting in a higher prevalence of precancerous lesions, gum loss, and loss of tooth structure next to the area of the cheek where the wad of tobacco is held. Baseball players are famous for the wad of tobacco many carry around in their mouths. These athlete-addicts have influenced many young people to copy their behavior and their addiction, often with the false belief that ST can enhance their athletic performance and that it's safe. Research has shown that ST has no effect on performance, and we've known for many years how immensely dangerous it is to keep a wad of tobacco pressed against your cheek.

Fortunately, the use of ST has been banned by virtually all of the well-known children's baseball organizations, as well as all of the minor league clubs. But as a recent article in the *Journal of the American Dental Association* said, "Even though dipping and chewing (of tobacco) is illegal on tens of thousands of diamonds across the country, its presence on just 28 major league diamonds undermines all the efforts."

As for smoking, we all are familiar with its dangers and how it greatly increases the risk of contracting cancer and heart disease. As if that isn't enough, it is also associated with adult gum disease and early-onset juvenile gum disease. The overwhelming conclusions of dental studies of smokers is that "the risk of smoking could greatly accelerate tooth loss."

The Special Needs of Older Dental Patients

This century has seen the life expectancy of Americans nearly double, from forty-six to about eighty. This increase has brought about a new focus on health problems of the elderly. Modern dentistry enables people to keep their mouths healthy, comfortable, and functioning. But for a variety of reasons this does not always apply to the elderly. Many elderly Americans are financially better off than other segments of our society, and dental care is a major source of financial outlay for them. Unfortunately, much of this dentistry may be substandard or unnecessary, leaving the patient with more serious and costly problems. Dr. Poorwork is particularly careless with the elderly, possibly calculating that they won't be around long enough to complain when the dentistry fails.

Some older patients who, throughout their lifetimes, have kept their mouths immaculately clean and enjoyed excellent oral health, suddenly begin to have serious problems of decay and periodontal disease. The cause almost always is a loss of skill and ability in toothbrushing. Although these patients may brush several times a day, because of loss of motor skills the brushing is ineffective. Other elderly patients may suffer depression or lack of motivation, again resulting in a falling down of effective oral hygiene. Moreover, others may suffer from any of the many diseases associated with aging; some of these diseases can affect the mouth directly, while others affect the ability to brush teeth correctly. Poor-quality dentistry that is maintained intact by meticulous oral hygiene will start to deteriorate as soon as the level of home care decreases. Bad dentistry is like a time bomb, waiting to go off when the fuse of incomplete cleaning is lit.

Complicating the loss of oral hygiene skills is a decrease in the amount of saliva. Saliva decreases as we get older. This situation can be aggravated by side effects from medications, poor diet, and systemic diseases such as diabetes and anemia. Saliva in the younger person helps keep the mouth clean and dilutes the harmful acids produced by the oral bacteria from food residue. The older person, now not brushing effectively, has much more food residue in the mouth but less saliva to neutralize it.

This new area of dentistry, concerned with the dental needs of the elderly, has been named "geriatric dentistry." Although this is not a specialty recognized by the American Dental Association, it is a valid area for those with a special interest and expertise, and there is even an American Society for Geriatric Dentistry. Topics that are being investigated include the relationship of osteoporosis to oral bone loss, root decay prevention, oral cancer detection, new methods of tooth cleaning, and chemotherapeutic (medicinal) methods of decay control and periodontal disease treatment.

Currently, the best approach is to use electric mechanical toothbrushes, which make it far easier to clean the teeth effectively, and fluoride mouthwashes, which increase the resistance to decay. A fluoride-containing chewing gum will soon be available. Chlorhexidine mouthwashes, available only by prescription, help fight plaque and bleeding gums, and help maintain periodontal health. The dentist can work with the patient's physician to find drugs that will not cause excessive oral dryness and to diagnose depression and nutritional deficiencies.

Although there is no completely satisfactory answer to this problem, the situation demands that the dentist change his normal treatment routine for such a patient. A dentist of conscience will not undertake to do a complex, heroic, and expensive program of treatment for a patient who is unable to brush properly and whose mouth is falling apart. Rather, the dentist is likely to focus on relieving pain and patching things as best as possible. Instead of a crown, the dentist may try a large filling, perhaps even a filling made of a less durable material that has pain-relieving properties. An ethical dentist is much more prone to treat very early cavities and slightly broken fillings, to keep them from rapidly deteriorating. When senior citizens who relocate to a retirement community go to a new dentist they may be told they need extensive dentistry. Caution is indicated; they should speak to the old dentist and get a second opinion. A nearby dental school is a good place to go for an unbiased exam.

We always tell our patients that going to the dentist is one of life's great pleasures, but we suspect that as people age this is one pleasure they would prefer to forgo. Although we may be unable to avoid problems with our teeth as we age, we can lower our risks by making sure the dentistry undergone at a younger age is properly done, that we maintain good oral hygiene, and that we avoid unnecessary dental treatment.

INFECTION CONTROL IN THE DENTIST'S OFFICE

In September 1990, Dr. David Acer, a dentist in Florida, died of AIDS. One of his patients, a young woman, was found to be infected with HIV, and it was also found by genetic testing, that at least five other patients had been infected by Dr. Acer. To this day he remains the only health-care worker ever determined to have passed the virus to his patients, though we still don't know how.

Theories abound. An editorial in *The New York Times* claimed that Dr. Acer was innocent and that his patients got infected because of their own dangerous and unreported behaviors. Another group declared that the transmission was through contaminated dental instruments. And several TV programs aired stories alleging that Dr. Acer, a homosexual, purposely infected his patients in order to bring publicity to the plight of AIDS-infected homosexuals. (The Centers for Disease Control could not find any evidence that Dr. Acer had purposely contaminated his syringes, and none of his staff ever saw him sticking himself with a needle. In fact, Dr. Acer's staff said he was very careful about sterilization and always wore gloves.)

Another theory is that Dr. Acer had an extremely contagious form of the virus for some period of time and unintentionally transmitted the disease. The other deadly bloodborne virus, hepatitis, has been transmitted by physicians in operating rooms, working under the most stringent infection controls. Although HIV is much less infective than hepatitis, it may be possible that it can be transmitted in this manner. But Acer's is the *only documented case* where AIDS was transmitted from health worker to patient.

In any case, Americans have entered a time of AIDS hysteria. People are afraid to go to their dentist or have an operation in a hospital. Nail salons and barbershops are suspect. So it's imperative that you know the facts and the risks of contracting disease at a dental office.

Fortunately, HIV is difficult to get. The risk of contracting it in everyday life, even if you have daily contact with AIDS patients, is minuscule. Furthermore, there has never been a documented case of cross-contamination, that is, infection being transferred from one patient to another by dental equipment, so you're safe in a dental office that also sees HIV-infected people. Yet patients are aware of the enormous efforts to "sterilize" the dental environment, and dentists are required by law to fulfill many time-consuming and expensive infection-control mandates. The ADA surveyed the dental community and estimated that the average per-year cost of infection control, per dentist, in a normal practice is $45,718.

The scientific information leads to the conclusion that the risk of transmission of HIV from patient to patient in a dental practice is zero, and the risk from dentist to patient and vice versa, if one of them has the virus, is extremely small.

Considering this, what course should we take? Dentists and other health care workers are legally required to work on all patients without taking any special steps for those with HIV (that's why gloves and masks are worn for all patients); this is called universal precautions. Health-care providers who are infected with HIV are not required to tell their patients. Being HIV positive is legally defined as a "disability" in order to protect those individuals from discrimination. Some argue that it is impossible to control this disease without proper public health measures, such as tracking the incidence and infective route of the virus. But this is precluded by a law that allows only AIDS cases, not HIV cases, to be reported. Since it may take as long as fifteen years for patients with HIV to develop AIDS, the transmission history of the virus cannot be determined. This leads to potentially dangerous gaps in our knowledge.

There are many sides to this complex issue. For example, it is possible to be HIV positive without knowing it, and the argument is made for mandatory testing so that the disease can be tracked. But even an accurate test may provide a great many false positives, and someone getting a false positive for HIV can suffer greatly as a result.

The general lack of knowledge about the disease also allows quacks to promote bogus treatments to "strengthen the immune system," thus implying that you will be less likely to get AIDS if you buy whatever the quack is selling. This can be deadly, because the false sense of security could lead to dangerous behavior such as unprotected sex or sharing of needles. Some dentists even tell their patients that the immune system can be improved by replacing all of their silver fillings or by wearing a plastic appliance or by taking a lot of unnecessary and overpriced food supplements. Don't fall for this nonsense. There is nothing a dentist can do for you or sell to you that will decrease your susceptibility to systemic, nonoral disease.

In any case, be assured that the risks associated with avoiding dental treatment due to fears of disease transmission are far greater than the risks of getting any disease in the dentist's office.

NUTRITION AND ORAL HEALTH

Proper nutrition affects the entire body, including the teeth—and it should begin early. When a baby is born, his teeth are already developing out-of-sight below the gums. Teeth usually start to develop during the seventh week of pregnancy. Pregnant women should ingest enough calcium, 1,200 mg. or about a quart of milk a day, to ensure adequate supplies for tooth development. The old wives' story that "my baby destroyed my teeth by taking the calcium out of them while I was pregnant" is false. If there's not enough calcium in the diet, the fetus will fulfill its requirements by taking calcium from the mother's bones, not from her teeth.

Vitamin D is also required for proper enamel formation, but take care not to overdose. Excessive vitamin D can cause a loss of appetite, headaches, nausea, diarrhea, fatigue, and other dangerous side effects.

Women who have severe nutritional deficiencies during pregnancy have an increased risk of having children with cleft lip and cleft palate. Fortunately, most nutrition-related diseases in the United States are due to overabundance, not deficiency, and therefore it is rare, except in the case of alcoholic or drug-addicted mothers, to see any severe deficiency diseases.

Fluoride, the most effective antidecay measure we have, is extremely important for young children. It is not known if fluoride passes through the placenta to the developing baby, but it is known that once the baby is born, fluoride will lead to substantial reductions in decay.

Women should avoid tetracycline antibiotics during pregnancy because they can affect fetal tooth development, causing permanent discoloration of the baby's teeth. Tetracyclines given to a young child can also lead to discoloration of the permanent teeth.

At the present time, the role of nutrition in the development and/or treatment of periodontal disease is unknown. Current research suggests that certain foods and nutrients can affect susceptibility to periodontal disease. It is thought that a well-balanced diet indirectly helps by keeping the mouth healthy and more resistant to the bacterial toxins that are a factor in both gum disease and decay.

Anorexia nervosa and bulimia are life-threatening eating disorders that often have oral symptoms. Patients with bulimia force themselves to vomit, sometimes several times a day, bathing the teeth in stomach acids that dissolve the enamel. Of course these patients have far more serious problems than enamel loss. The excessive weight loss associated with these diseases can cause fatal chemical imbalances. Dentists can often diagnose these conditions by noting the acid-eroded teeth.

Severe vitamin C deficiency leads to a disease called scurvy. Its symptoms include reddened, inflamed, bleeding gums, a dry mouth, and the eventual loosening and loss of teeth. There have been cases of people who take large daily doses of vitamin C getting "rebound scurvy" if they stop taking the vitamin too quickly. Vitamin C chemically is ascorbic acid and, because it's an acid, chewing tablets of C can cause the enamel to dissolve.

Vitamin B deficiency can lead to inflammation of the corners of the mouth, called angular chelitis, and inflammation of the tongue, called glossitis. This is sometimes seen on older patients who are not eating well. A caution: Almost everybody gets enough nutritional elements from ordinary eating. In America most people taking supplements don't need them. Taking extra vitamins and other supplements is almost never necessary, and can do harm. Vitamins and other food supplements should be taken only to treat a diagnosed insufficiency, which, in well-fed America, is rare.

Good nutrition, a balanced diet, meticulous oral hygiene, and fluoride can, along with appropriate dental care, usually assure a lifetime of good oral health.

AUXILIARY DENTAL PERSONNEL

The intelligent use of well-trained auxiliaries is a must in modern practice. There are three categories: dental assistants, dental hygienists, and dental laboratory technicians.

Dental Assistants

The duties of dental assistants vary from state to state, but in general, they seat and prepare patients, sterilize instruments, prepare materials, keep records, develop X rays, and use the high-volume suction while the dentist is drilling. Many assistants receive their training on-the-job at the dentist's office while others take a commercial course or receive special instruction for expanded duties, such as taking X rays. Additional training is required to become a registered dental assistant (RDA). RDAs are legally permitted to polish teeth and in some states are allowed to apply sealants.

Dental Hygienists

Dental hygienists usually have a two-year A.A. degree or four-year B.A. in dental hygiene. They become registered by passing a state licensing exam. The scope of what hygienists can do varies from state to state, but they routinely clean and polish the teeth, take and develop X rays, examine teeth for decay and gums for periodontal disease, and teach oral health care.

We feel that many of the problems blossoming in the coming days of managed care could be satisfactorily solved by the expanded and intelligent use of assistants and hygienists. These auxiliaries can be trained to competently perform more dental procedures than they are now permitted to do. For example, working under the supervision of a dentist, a trained auxiliary should be able to fill teeth and take impressions on teeth prepared by the dentist. The dentist should do the diagnosis and treatment planning, and execute procedures deemed too difficult for the auxiliaries. If managed care clinics of the future, instead of compelling their dentists to work much faster, utilize trained auxiliaries in expanded functions, costs can be lowered without degrading the quality of service.

There need be no anxiety on the part of the public about allowing nondentists to perform dentistry. We would much prefer a trained, dentist-supervised auxiliary to fill our teeth than Dr. Poorwork.

Dental Laboratory Technicians

Dental laboratory technicians are trained to construct and repair fixed and removable dental restorations such as crowns, inlays, and dentures. Their work is done away from the patient using impressions taken on the patient by the dentist. Most learn by being apprenticed, but others have up to a year of commercial school training. Almost all dental technicians work under the direction of a dentist, although a few states have passed laws allowing technicians to market dentures directly to the public.

There are Poorwork dental laboratories, which don't take the care and time needed to do accurate work. Dr. Poorwork always deals with these labs because they are cheap. But don't worry; Dr. Goodwork doesn't use these labs and pays considerably more for a lab doing the work right. Conversely, at times Dr. Poorwork sends work to a good-quality lab, hoping for a better-looking result. But the good lab doesn't know what to do with Poorwork's sloppy preparations and slipshod impressions! So the Poorwork dentists and the Poorwork labs find each other and stay together.

For many years a small group of dental laboratory technicians, calling themselves denturists, have lobbied the government to be allowed to market full dentures directly to the public, without having a dentist oversee the entire process. They argue that patients seeking full dentures have no teeth, dentists charge "too much" for the rather simple process of making a denture, and the lab technician actually makes the denture, often with little or no supervision or instruction other than tooth color. Therefore, they propose that a lab technician could make just as good a full denture as a dentist and for much less money. In some ways their argument has merit: At times dentures can be a rather straightforward and uncomplicated service. Some state legislatures have bowed to this argument and have passed laws allowing the direct marketing of dentures to the public.

We strongly disagree. It is imperative that the patient be carefully and expertly examined. Even though no teeth may be involved, there can still be oral infections, tumors, and other diseases and conditions that lab technicians are not trained to identify, let alone treat. Ignoring these could be potentially deadly. Also, in many cases the mouth needs special treatments in order for a full denture to fit properly (see Chapter 14). In these cases, the technician is not qualified to evaluate the patient and provide appropriate treatment.

The job of laboratory technician is highly diverse and requires considerable training in many complex procedures. It makes no sense to require a technician also to study the whole medical phase of a dentist's training. This is the background a technician would need in order to diagnose oral disease. Even Dr. Poorwork can recognize severe disease, such as oral cancer, and refer the patient for treatment. But denturists do not have the necessary training.

7. Pain and Emergency Treatments

*

PAIN

For most people, if we say the word "dentistry," it is likely that the first word that comes to mind is "pain." This is understandable, not only because of the legendary image of the dentist as a pain purveyor but also because of the very sensitive nature of the mouth. The teeth and gums can be a source of pain ranging from mild to excruciating, from occasional to chronic.

Dental pain can ruin the pleasures of eating and even keep one up at night. It can be an annoying twinge or a full-blown toothache. In the good-quality practice, episodes of patient pain are rare; well-kept and well-treated mouths almost never experience toothache. But Dr. Poorwork's patients are often in pain and suffer the consequences—extractions, which are the quickest (but not the best) way to eliminate tooth pain.

The dental pulp, the tissue inside the tooth, is the most common source of severe pain. It is often called "the nerve," but it is really a highly vascular (blood-filled) and extremely sensitive tissue. A condition of slight and reversible irritation of the pulp is called hyperemia. The hyperemic tooth is sensitive to cold and, sometimes, to the action of food juices or sugary or acidic drinks. The pain could come and go, disappearing entirely for long periods of time and returning for brief episodes that sometimes conform to the change of seasons, when heightened anxiety can increase blood pressure slightly, making the pulp more sensitive. Most of us have experienced certain days when teeth have reacted to cold foods such as ice cream.

More serious, irreversible pain is called pulpitis, characterized by strong reactions to biting pressure or heat, or at worst, a constant, acute toothache. This is commonly caused by extensive decay, when the bacteria penetrate to the root canal and infect the pulp. The pulp, like any infected tissue, tends to swell, but, unlike other tissues, the pulp is confined within the hard walls of the tooth and has no place to swell. The resulting pressures that build up can cause excruciating pain. Pulpitis can also occur as a result of a blow to the tooth, the toxic irritation of poorly insulated filling materials, or even overenthusiastic drilling by a dentist.

The gums can be a source of pain—from infections, developing wisdom teeth, denture sores, and many other causes. The important thing to remember is that mouth pain is the sign of a real, not psychosomatic, ailment that should be diagnosed and corrected. Sometimes the diagnosis is hard to pinpoint, but we have never seen a case of what we could call imaginary mouth pain. Dr. Poorwork, not taking the time to do a thorough examination, might call the patient's pain emotional. "She's a nut!" he complains. Dr. Goodwork knuckles down and takes the time necessary to make a better diagnosis. And Dr. Quack might blame it on allergies or other bizarre causes instead of actually diagnosing the true cause.

Mild discomfort following some dental procedures is common; occasionally the patient leaves the office feeling worse than when he came in. A deep periodontal scaling can cause some pain later on or even the next day. A newly filled tooth can be sensitive to cold for up to a few weeks (because the deep metal filling can conduct temperature change deep into the tooth, or perhaps because deep drilling slightly inflamed the pulp, or because of a reaction to the filling material.) But serious postoperative pain is rare. A rule of thumb is that if the pain cannot be controlled by an over-the-counter painkiller like aspirin, Advil, or Tylenol, then call the dentist. (Responsible dentists always leave a telephone number where they or a covering dentist can be reached in an emergency. Even after office hours, the good dentist leaves a forwarding number on the answering machine. One of the characteristics of many Poorworks is the absence of this service.)

Occasionally a new filling comes into contact with an older filling, causing a pain called a galvanic reaction. This is because no two fillings made at different times have exactly the same metallic proportions, and when different metal alloys come into contact, a mild electric current may be generated, causing slight pain. Usually these episodes of galvanic pain disappear after a few days.

Traumatic occlusion can cause postoperative symptoms. Occlusion (also called the "bite") refers to the way the teeth fit when the jaws come together. If a filling is left too high, that tooth comes into premature contact with its opposing tooth every time the patient closes his jaws. That tooth, by itself taking a blow usually shared by the rest of the teeth, often becomes sensitive. The dentist can easily correct this by grinding down the high spot of the filling.

Many people put off needed dental visits because of fear of pain. But today the great majority of dental procedures can be accomplished entirely without pain. The local anesthetics used today, derived from the classic Novocain, are marvelously efficient and safe. While the injection might hurt a little, it is rarely very painful, and the benefits to the patient in freedom from pain, and to the dentist in being able to work on a relaxed and cooperative patient, cannot be overestimated.

A more recent method of local anesthesia is the intraligamental injection. In this technique, used mostly for the lower jaw, a small amount of anesthetic is injected into the periodontal ligament that attaches the tooth to the jaw. The needle is placed right into the gum alongside the root of the tooth. Some patients find this type of injection to be painless, while others complain that it hurts. (It may depend on the thickness of the individual's periodontal ligament.) Its major advantage is that it usually doesn't hurt, numbs only the tooth being treated, and lasts only for an hour. (The block injection on the lower jaw often hurts somewhat and numbs all the lower teeth on that side for up to four hours.) The major drawback of the intraligamental injection is that it doesn't always work: perhaps 10 percent of the time it is not effective, and then we have to use the block injection anyway.

There are other methods of controlling pain and anxiety. Premedication can calm anxious patients. Some dentists work with general anesthesia, putting the patient entirely to sleep. Others use nitrous oxide gas ("laughing gas"), which supplies partial anesthesia. But we feel that local anesthesia administered by injection is by far the best and most convenient method for use in the dental office.

Dentistry done under general anesthesia involves a troubling conflict of interest. As we have repeatedly stated, adequate time is the essential element in performing quality dentistry. But when the patient is under general anesthesia, speed is imperative; the less time the patient is unconscious the safer the procedure. So the dentist is torn between taking the time needed for a quality result and protecting the safety of the patient. We feel that general anesthesia in dentistry should be reserved for patients with serious physical infirmity (for example, seizure disorders) or uncontrollable phobias that make conventional treatment impossible.

A variety of gimmicks have been used to reduce pain, usually without success. Electronic analgesia units deliver a small electric "shock" to the patient. The intensity and frequency of the shocks are controlled by the patient, and it is claimed that the device often eliminates the need for injections. A recent study detected no improvement in pain on patients treated with these devices or with a placebo device. Transcutaneous electric neural stimulation (TENS) units have also been shown to be ineffective in treating pain. Hypnotism, acupuncture, other electronic contraptions, herbs—none of these has been proved effective except perhaps for the placebo effect and the patient's suggestibility. Don't waste your time or money buying or renting one of these devices. (See Chapter 20.)

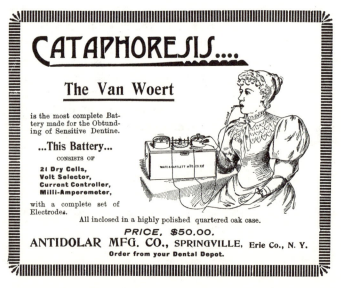

This is an ad from an 1897 dental journal promoting an early form of electrical anesthesia. Cataphoresis, as it was then called, didn't work and was not adopted by the dental profession. TENS and electro-anesthesia are direct descendants of this device and don't appear to work any better. (Illustration from *Items of Interest,* A Monthly Magazine of Dental Art, Science and Literature, January 1897.)

A variety of facial pain recently has received considerable publicity. Assumed by some to be related to the jaw joints, it is generally called TMJ after the *temporomandibular joint*. This type of pain can be serious, even debilitating, and is very difficult to treat. Most of the information foisted on the public about this condition has at best been anecdotal speculation and at worst the self-serving lies of quacks. Effective treatments include simple painkillers, anti-inflammatory and antidepressant drugs, "trigger point" injections, and, especially, exercises. But other common treatments, including reshaping the bite with appliances or fixed bridgework or grinding the teeth, biofeedback, acupuncture, kinesiology, vitamins, electrical stimulators, and chiropractic are useless except for the placebo effect. (Chapter 20 provides extensive detail on this subject.)

Some patients exhibit an extreme sensitivity to the slightest changes in their bite. A dentist who fails to diagnose this situation and attempts to adjust or rebuild the bite is merely going to produce more serious trouble for the patient.

The cracked tooth presents another difficult-to-diagnose problem. A tooth can crack and be sensitive each time the patient bites down in a particular way; over a period of time the crack can get deeper until the tooth is split lengthwise and must be extracted. Thus, early diagnosis is important—but difficult. New methods of diagnosing cracks have been developed, and the intraoral TV can be a big help, enabling the dentist to see a greatly magnified view of an otherwise most difficult-to-see tooth surface. Once the diagnosis is made, the tooth can be treated by making a crown, which holds the tooth together, preventing the crack from widening.

EMERGENCY DENTAL TREATMENTS

This section addresses those emergencies that we've been called about (usually on a Sunday morning) and tells you what to do if you can't get to a dentist.

Broken tooth. If it doesn't hurt, you can wait for a normal dental visit. If the tooth is sharp, you can cover the sharp edge with some wax and see your dentist as soon as possible. Sometimes, if the sharp point is cutting your tissues, you can smooth it off *slightly* with an emery board or a fine file, but this has some risk unless done carefully. Drugstores also carry over-the-counter temporary filling materials. You can use some cotton with Vaseline on it to cover the tooth until a professional repair can be done.

Toothache. A toothache needs prompt professional attention. Anti-inflammatory drugs such as aspirin or ibuprofen lessen the pain, but a tooth that hurts needs a dentist—pain is a sign of a problem. Some people believe that it's good to put aspirin directly on the gum near the offending tooth, but *this is wrong.* Aspirin, an acid, can burn and severely irritate the gum tissue. Sometimes the pain is caused by food stuck between the teeth, and simple flossing and rinsing with warm salt water solves the problem. If the pain is severe and the tooth reacts to heat and to pressure, try ice or a cold can of soda on the cheek near the painful tooth and get to a dentist as soon as possible. If a tooth has been acting up, with some pain on and off, avoid vigorous exercise, flying, or scuba diving. Activity and change of external pressures can cause a delicate pulp to go over the edge and deliver acute pain.

Teething. Children often complain of pain when their baby teeth are coming in, or when the baby teeth are getting loose and being replaced by the permanent teeth. Symptoms include red, swollen gums, excessive drooling, a slightly elevated temperature, crankiness, and not being able to sleep. A frozen reusable teething ring is very useful as are over-the-counter medications such as Tylenol. But remember, you should never give a child medicine that is prescribed for adults, even if it's only one-half or one-fourth of a dosage. We recommend against using topical anesthetics because they taste terrible and can also anesthetize the child's tongue and throat. Some people recommend rubbing whisky on the gum because the alcohol may have a slight anesthetic action; we think little of this method.

Displaced or knocked-out tooth. A tooth can be knocked out in a sporting accident or a fight. Try to find the tooth, put it in a wet cloth (putting it in ice water is excellent) and get to your dentist or hospital emergency room immediately. A tooth can be put back into the original socket, but speed is essential.

Swelling. A swollen gum or cheek is almost always a sign of infection and requires immediate attention. Don't ever put yourself on antibiotics and wait to see if they work. Get to a dentist or an emergency room!

Canker sores. It's estimated that over half the population will have a canker sore at one time or another. Although they heal within two weeks, they can be extremely unpleasant, and some people have recurrent episodes of canker sores. Canker sores are usually found on the inside of the cheek or on the tongue and are often caused by biting or burning the mouth while eating. Ice and topical anesthetics are useful. Chlorhexidine mouthwash has been found to be helpful in treatment.

Avoid irritating the canker sore with spicy acidic foods such as salad dressing or orange juice. If the canker sore hasn't disappeared within two weeks, contact your dentist.

Tooth grinding. Grinding the teeth while sleeping is called bruxism and is thought to be a genetic trait. About 20 percent of the population grinds. Contrary to popular belief, chronic bruxism rarely causes the teeth to wear down, nor does it lead to TMJ. Tooth grinding does seem to be triggered in susceptible people by anxiety. No treatment is necessary unless the enamel is wearing down or there is pain.

TMJ, Jaw Pain, or Locked Jaw. If you can move your jaw, use alternating hot and cold compresses, two or three minutes per application, don't chew hard food or gum, don't open your mouth wide, be careful of yawning, move the jaw gently from side to side, and take ibuprofen (Advil). If your jaw has locked, try to relax and place a warm moist compress over the jaw joint (in front of the ear), take ibuprofen, and after a half hour try *gently* to open the mouth, wiggling gently from side to side. If it's still stuck, see a dentist or go to an emergency room. Once your jaw starts to work again, go easy on chewing and opening wide for a few weeks. TMJ has been a fertile field for the quacks. (See Chapter 20.)

Wisdom Teeth. A painful inflammation, usually infectious, can develop around the crown of an erupting tooth, usually a wisdom tooth. Most wisdom teeth are at least partially impacted, that is, "stuck" in the jaw because there is not enough room for them to emerge fully. In such cases, with the tooth half in and half out, a flap of gum tissue is produced. This flap is a marvelous food trap and source of infection. These infections can become quite serious and should be treated promptly. Warning signs include pain and swelling in the area of the wisdom tooth and difficulty opening the mouth, especially in the morning. Warm salt-water rinses help clean the area and possibly help draw out the infection. The ultimate treatment for recurrent infection of this type is usually the removal of the impacted wisdom tooth; as a temporary treatment, the dentist may establish drainage for the infection and cleanse the area.

8. The Examination and the Dentist's Tools

*

I t goes without saying that proper dental treatment cannot be accomplished without a thorough examination. This examination provides the information the dentist must have to develop a diagnosis and a plan of treatment, and then to inform the patient of possible options and approximate fees (of course the examination fee should be quoted beforehand).

The clinical examination is conducted with the eyes, fingers, instruments, and diagnostic aids. The dentist looks carefully at the bones, teeth, gums, cheeks, tongue, palate, and floor of mouth, using a dental mirror to retract structures and to reflect light on difficult-to-see areas. With the fingers the dentist feels the tissues, particularly any swollen, irritated areas or lesions. He also feels for tooth movement and looseness. Explorers can be used to check for surface cavities and loose or poor-fitting fillings and crowns, and periodontal probes check for the existence and severity of pockets at the gum line. Special plastic biting instruments are used to diagnose cracked teeth. And some dentists have closed-circuit television cameras capable of taking and showing pictures intraorally. This expensive gadget is quite useful for diagnosis and patient education, but it can also be used by Dr. Fraud to sell unnecessary dental work. (We talk more about this when we come to other dental machinery.)

X RAYS

X rays, discovered in 1895, have become a necessary part of a dental examination. Without them a dentist cannot detect early decay, bone loss of periodontal disease, developmental abnormalities, retained roots, impacted teeth, tumors, cysts, infections, and other diseases and abnormalities. An examination without X rays is like reading with closed eyes. An initial adult examination generally requires fourteen to sixteen separate X rays. Depending on the patient, such a complete exam need be done only every five to ten years. Every two or three years a smaller, "bite-wing" series, which checks for mouthwide decay and gum disease, should be enough.

The concept of quality also applies to examination and X rays. A good examination takes time, which Poorwork is not willing to take. And Dr. Poorwork often uses unqualified, unlicensed, even illegal personnel to take X rays, or if he takes them himself he does it carelessly. To be of value, X rays should be carefully set up and positioned, with exact exposure and development time. Many Poorworks take X rays just to get the fee, while their sloppy X rays have little diagnostic value.

Some dentists use a panoramic X-ray machine, which takes a view of the entire mouth with one large film and uses less radiation. The resulting film shows the teeth, roots, and any pathological structures in exact relationship to each other, and is appropriate and very useful for oral surgeons and orthodontists. We feel, however, that panoramic X rays do not provide the exact details of decay, infected bone structure, and periodontal attachment that are crucial to problems encountered by general dentists, periodontists, and endodontists, and therefore should not be used by these latter groups.

X rays are one of the dentist's diagnostic tools and must remain with him as part of his records. But any reputable dentist will make X rays and other records available to any other dentist if the patient so requests.

The risks of X rays have been highly exaggerated. Today X-ray films are amazingly fast and require a tiny fraction of the radiation exposure previously needed. When Dr. Schissel first entered practice it was customary for dentists to take X rays every six months, and the radiation per exposure was nearly twenty times the amount used today. One single X ray taken then required more radiation exposure than a full initial set of sixteen X rays requires today. Even so, responsible dentists today use X rays only at two- or three-year intervals or when necessary for emergency diagnosis.

Standard safety measures should be followed. Patients should be covered with a lead apron when X rays are taken. The X-ray machine should be fitted with an open-ended plastic cylinder rather than a cone, because this means that the amount of radiation has been properly focused and reduced by almost half. The dentist should be using "E-speed" film (the fastest film available at this writing, requiring half the exposure time of the older "D-speed" film). With modern equipment and technique, dental X rays are completely safe for all patients, including children and pregnant women.

HISTORY TAKING

Careful history taking is essential, especially in these days of an aging population taking many medications. The dentist must not only find out what work has been done in the mouth but also get a careful record of the patient's physical condition and medications used. Allergic reactions to drugs, and medical conditions such as valvular heart problems that require antibiotic premedication, are examples of things that must be noted. The dentist must know whether root canal was done or attempted for a tooth, or if braces were ever worn; these might have a bearing on projected treatment. Additional diagnostic procedures, for example, study models or lab tests, may be needed for patients with special problems.

As with all other phases of good dentistry, a proper dental examination cannot be completed in a few minutes. A major part of the dentist's responsibility after completing the examination is to tell the patient, in nontechnical terms, what his oral condition is, what can be done, and what to expect if it is not done. The dentist can suggest alternative treatments and fees; sometimes the most desirable treatment is beyond the patient's means, and a less desirable but still satisfactory treatment is agreed upon. Of course, it is up to the reputable dentist to see that whatever treatment is adopted is sound. The patient's education does not stop here but is a continuing process and the never-ending responsibility of the dentist.

Such a thorough examination is not necessary at every checkup; recall checkups need not be so extensive. Depending on the patient, the nature of follow-up examinations and their frequency should be carefully considered by the dentist.

THE DRILL

Sometimes a dentist is judged more by the array of machinery in his shop than by his professional results. "I go to Dr. P. He has all the latest equipment."

The technological revolution of the last half century has inevitably involved dentistry, which depends heavily on machinery to achieve its results. A multitude of new approaches and styles in dental equipment have been developed. Most are simply variations on old ones, but some are significant improvements in ease of operation for the dentist and increased comfort for the patient. But shiny new equipment is no assurance that the dentistry performed with this equipment is competent or up-to-date. Sorry to say, much of today's old-fashioned, inadequate, and downright bad dentistry is done with brand-new equipment.

One word more than any other evokes horror and fear of the dentist—"the drill." The drill is the most valuable instrument in the dentist's office. Without it, the dentist is virtually helpless, unable to accomplish the most basic dentistry.

The dentist's drill consists of a machine that operates a rotary drill bit, which may be a bur, disk, grinding stone, or scaling or polishing device. These drill bits are used to remove decay and weak tooth structure, and to extend, groove, bevel, and shape teeth to receive restorations. It is needed to polish fillings and teeth and to adjust occlusion (bite)—in short, for every routine procedure.

Those old enough to have experienced dentistry with the old, slow, belt-driven drills remember the dentist "leaning" on the tooth, and the vibrations and rattling sensations of that drill. Modern high-speed drills are much smoother and easier. But at high speeds the heat of friction can become a problem. Excessive heat damages the pulp of a tooth, making the tooth sensitive and perhaps requiring root canal work. As a precaution, the high-speed drills use a water spray that cools the tooth during drilling. The dentist must also take care to avoid sustained pressure on any part of the tooth because this causes excess heat.

The so-called painless drills are anything but. Deep drilling without anesthesia can be excruciating. But shallow drilling and partial preparation of a decayed tooth can be done without pain. This is how some Dr. Poorworks get away without giving injections: They make a perfunctory pass at the tooth, removing some decay in a very short time but without properly preparing the tooth or cleaning out all the decay; then the tooth is filled. This way the patient is impressed with the quick and painless "no-needle" treatment, and may not wise up for years, until the ruinous results of Poorwork dentistry become apparent. And many patients never wise up, because they have been brainwashed into believing that it is natural for people to lose teeth as a matter of course and accept their loss of teeth without ever blaming Dr. Poorwork.

Many dentists feel that no drill operated at high speeds is suitable for the removal of deep decay, as this is partly a matter of "feel" in the hands of the dentist. Often there is no room for error, since there is only an extremely thin layer of sound tooth structure between the decay and the pulp. It is important to preserve this layer; if it is perforated, work on the tooth will be complicated by a root canal procedure. That is why most dentists switch to a slow-speed drill to complete removal of deep decay. But not Dr. Poorwork. His high-speed drill can remove some tooth structure painlessly, without the need for an injection. Poorwork's patients appreciate this, and also appreciate that when a slight pain is felt from the drilling, Poorwork stops and fills the tooth—right on top of the remaining decay.

OTHER DENTAL MACHINERY

The Cavitron is a type of handpiece that develops supersonic vibrations. Today it is used as an aid for periodontal scaling. The Cavitron (and its clones) can remove heavy deposits of tartar quickly and easily, thus saving the dentist considerable time. It's best to finish the scaling meticulously with hand scalers, though; the Cavitron is generally not considered adequate to do a complete and adequate scaling. But for mouths with heavy tartar it is a valuable time-saver.

The prophy-jet is a device that sprays a slightly abrasive solution on the tooth, easily removing stains. Although it can be useful, it can also take the polish off porcelain restorations and dull the finish of some fillings. It requires very careful use.

Some dentists are making use of the new and dramatic intraoral television. In this expensive technology, tiny TV cameras, designed to fit into the mouth, can photograph the most remote surfaces of the teeth. These cameras are connected to monitors and printers and can be hooked up to computers and tape recorders. This machinery can be helpful for diagnosis and even treatment, but it is used mostly for promotional purposes, to get the patient to accept what the dentist plans to do.

Using the TV, a dentist can show his patient a highly magnified picture, filling the TV screen, of a tooth. If the tooth is decayed or fractured, the lesion will appear very startling on the screen. Shocked by the magnified appearance of the lesion, the patient is more likely to accept the dentist's recommendations for proper treatment. This can be a big help to the ethical dentist, but Dr. Fraud can use this to panic the patient into having unnecessary work. Even a completely sound tooth can look frightening when greatly magnified.

Some dentists have this apparatus attached to a computer. When the picture of the patient's smile appears on the screen, the computer can manipulate the picture to show how gorgeous the patient will look after treatment—or at least how the dentist *thinks* the case will come out.

NEW GIMMICKS

Patients often complain about the sound of the drill, and a lot of research effort has been expended to develop silent drills. Lasers were tried, but they caused overheating and damage to the tooth. In the summer of 1996 the FDA Dental Products Advisory Committee rejected an application for a laser designed to "drill" teeth. The FDA cited a lack of evidence that the laser is effective and safe. High-frequency sound vibrations were also unsuccessful. Recently two other methods have been widely advertised: chemical dissolving of decay and using abrasives driven by air pressure. The chemical device, called CARIDAX, has not become popular; it is a slow process and still requires some drilling.

The newest, and not yet widely available method is a high-pressure stream of abrasive, similar to a sandblaster, to remove tooth structure. The promoters of these devices claim that anesthesia is usually not necessary, and that the method is faster, silent, and vibration free. The downside to this machine, in addition to its cost, which is passed on to the patient, is that it does not remove decay and is useful only for small, easily accessible cavities, many so small that they need not be treated at all. Another problem involves the use of alpha alumina particles as the abrasive. Both the patient and the dental staff are exposed to considerable airborne particles of alpha alumina, and there is insufficient data showing that these particles are safe to inhale.

LASERS

Lasers are a useful device in some fields of medicine, and there are some claimed uses for high-power lasers in dentistry. The high-power laser is used by some dentists to "cut" soft tissues, such as the gums, in effect replacing a scalpel, but the results are not convincing. The FDA has not approved high-power lasers for use on hard tissues such as bone or tooth, although some dentists are using these expensive devices for etching enamel, curing bonded fillings, and other nonapproved procedures. At this time we see little value or advantage in high-power lasers for dental use.

Some dentists and physical therapists claim that low-power lasers, the type in a CD player or supermarket checkout scanner, can be used as a penetrating source of heat to treat deep soreness and pain in muscles and joints, particularly in patients with TMJ. This approach has scant positive research to back it up, and it's much too early to endorse or use it.

Other dentists, however, have proposed a novel and vastly different application of the soft laser as a treatment for patients with all types of headaches. Possibly because they believe that most headaches are caused by something close to the mouth, they claim that it's appropriate for dentists to treat headache patients. One leading advocate of this method plays a low-power laser on the throat and claims to help migraine headaches. However, the scientific consensus at this time is that low-power lasers have no biologic effect whatsoever, and exploiting the hopes of migraine sufferers is a particularly repulsive quackery.

A more dangerous headache treatment is known as radiofrequency surgical cauterization (RSC). RSC does have some legitimate medical applications, but not to treat headaches. Recently, however, a number of dentists have started promoting the use of RSC to cure all headaches by destroying parts of three important tissues: the stylomandibular ligament, a tendon attaching a facial muscle to the skull, and a pair of nerves to muscles on the head. These are dangerous, experimental treatments outside the scope of dentistry.

9. Decay and Its Treatment

*

Tooth decay, or caries, is the most prevalent disease of all humanity, more common than the common cold. With caries so widespread, providing limitless opportunity for study, you might expect that we have learned all about this major scourge. We have indeed learned much, but its innermost secrets, like that of the cold, have so far eluded our investigations.

Present theory of the cause of decay involves bacteria, acids, dental plaque, food residue, salivary pH, and bad oral hygiene. The dental plaque, a composite of bacteria and food debris, is considered to play a major role in decay. But we don't know enough about the specific role played by any of these factors, and, except for the conventional methods of immaculate oral hygiene and the fluoridation of community water supplies, we haven't been able to develop a sure method of intercepting the decay process and preventing or curing the disease. We know that decay progresses at different rates in different environments. Some individuals, for a variety of reasons, experience rapid rates of tooth decay, while in other mouths decay proceeds very slowly. In some people a very small cavity doesn't change for years, while in others an identical lesion reaches serious proportions within a year. It is most likely, for instance, that decay proceeds apace in an acid medium. People whose saliva tends to be less acid are more resistant to decay, but they are more prone to tartar formation and resultant gum disease. These statements about saliva and decay are oversimplifications subject to some scientific reservations, but they nevertheless convey some idea of the relation of oral chemistry to tooth pathology.

Controversy exists concerning the effects of "bad habits" such as smoking, drinking, and drug use on oral health. Many experts condemn smoking, especially as a factor in periodontal disease. Alcohol and drug abuse are usually associated with poor oral hygiene and increased decay and gum problems.

The characteristics of saliva play a part in caries susceptibility.

Thick, heavy saliva tends to retain food residues and build up plaque. Some people have a thin, watery saliva that washes away food debris and reduces caries incidence. A person's diet is another factor. Diets high in processed sugars and other refined carbohydrates readily form tacky food residues that are hard to remove (plaque); with bacterial and enzymatic help, they quickly produce acid by-products that attack the teeth.

Thorough and prompt oral hygiene after eating sharply reduces the decay-producing potential of everything you eat and drink. It is the presence of these foods *in the mouth,* not in the stomach, that is dangerous. Diet is a factor in dental decay only as it is related to the efficiency of oral hygiene. Providing your child with fresh fruit and vegetables and other elements of a healthy diet "to build sound teeth" will not succeed unless the child also is taught effective oral hygiene. Another vital factor in cavity prevention is the inclusion of fluoride in the diet. Children who drink fluoride-free bottled water "because it is healthier" are much more susceptible to decaying teeth.

Even severe childhood nutritional deficiencies rarely affect the teeth. Nature gives priority to the developing dentition. A calcium deficiency in a child can result in rickets, a disease of the bones, but it almost never affects the calcification of the teeth. Ignorance about oral hygiene and poor dental treatment are to blame for diseased or lost teeth, not early poverty and parents who failed to provide a proper diet.

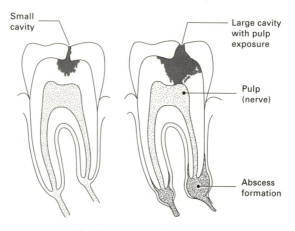

Small cavity

Large cavity with pulp exposure

Pulp (nerve)

Abscess formation

The Progress of Decay

Control of diet in young children is especially important because children do not have sufficient manual dexterity or self-discipline to maintain effective oral hygiene. Many children show a pattern of "continuous eating"; they are always chewing on fruit, bread, or lollipops. Since continuous brushing is not feasible, an attempt should be made to control the child's diet, especially eliminating foods that promote decay. Hard sucking candies, for example, produce a sugary acid component in the saliva for long periods of time. There is nothing worse than a lollipop for a caries-prone child. Sugary chewing gum and soda pop are other serious offenders.

The role of heredity in caries is not understood. While a son may seemingly "inherit" his dad's buckteeth, bad gums, or decay-prone teeth, it is likely that learned chewing habits, learned habits of oral hygiene and learned attitudes about dental treatment are more important. And the services of Dr. Poorwork can be passed from parent to child. It might be noted that, although the amount of tooth decay in Americans has decreased significantly because of fluoridation, American children from minority groups, rural areas, those with minimal exposure to fluoride, and those from less-educated and less-affluent families have a much higher incidence of cavities.

Though the teeth of some people are constitutionally more disposed to the ravages of decay than the teeth of more fortunate others, it is more accurate to say that some *mouths* are more prone to decay than others, and for many reasons (chemistry, saliva, oral hygiene, and so on). There is no longer any doubt that teeth with more fluoride in their composition are considerably more resistant to decay than those with less fluoride. But there is no such thing as "soft teeth"; *all* teeth are *very* hard. In fact, tooth enamel is much harder than iron, gold, and porcelain. The expression "soft teeth" is often used erroneously to refer to teeth with many cavities. This term is often taken literally by the patient, who despairs of ever being able to keep his teeth and who resigns himself to early dentures. "Soft teeth" is a favorite expression of Dr. Poorwork to explain why his work so often "goes bad." Of course, *his* patients have every reason to despair about the future of their teeth, but not because they are soft.

FILLINGS

The treatment of dental caries can be generally summed up in the rule: Remove decay completely and restore the teeth to form and function. Of course this is easier said than done. Removal of the decay, although a difficult and delicate job, is the simpler task. And we mean *complete* removal of decay. For years some dentists, particularly the Poorworks, have maintained that it is not necessary to remove all decay; that the lowest layer of decay is sterile and will remain inactive if the tooth is carefully sealed by the filling. This has been the theoretical justification for Dr. Poorwork's refusal to take the time necessary to clean out a cavity thoroughly. But it is not true; the lowest layer of decay *is* bacteriologically active and *does* cause recurrent decay. Good dentists have always known this, and scientific studies have confirmed it.

The restorative considerations and work can be exceedingly complex. Usually a tooth can be saved even if only a sound root stump remains. (If so little is left of the root that extraction is the only solution, the missing tooth is replaced.) If the tooth is restorable, but the caries involves the pulp, then root canal work is usually required. If the crown of the tooth is badly broken down, then a full crown or large cast restoration is needed. Finally, if the decay has not done major damage, treatment is the most common dental restoration, the filling. (Let us be clear that a cavity is a carious lesion, a defect, a hole in a tooth, something that must be corrected, while the filling is the treatment or correction of the defect. These two terms often get confused.)

The steps in the preparation and construction of a silver-amalgam filling are outlined in Chapter 5. Essentially: (1) all decay and any weakened tooth structure are removed; (2) the remaining tooth structure is shaped and/or prepared chemically to hold the filling material, insulate the tooth, and minimize the possibility of future decay at that site; and (3) the filling is then carefully placed in the tooth. These procedures take time, but a properly made filling may last indefinitely, while a badly made filling almost invariably fails.

Many materials have been used to make fillings, including various metals, cements, porcelains, and plastics, but dentistry still does not have a perfect restorative material. To be absolutely perfect, a filling material must have many important qualities:

- It should be aesthetic. It should look exactly like part of the tooth that was replaced, both in form and color.
- It must be nonpoisonous.
- It must be readily manipulable in the mouth. High-fusing porcelain looks good and makes an excellent material for some types of fillings, but since it must be baked at temperatures well over one thousand degrees Fahrenheit, it cannot be used for fillings that are to be shaped in the mouth.
- It must be resistant to abrasion, both from the wear of chewing and at contact points with neighboring teeth.
- The material must be stable. A filling must not dissolve in or react chemically with anything likely to enter the mouth. It must not break down with temperature changes or the passage of time.
- It must have good crushing and edge strength. The forces of chewing are tremendous. A filling must be resistant to breaking, crushing, and chipping.
- The material, once placed in the cavity, should not flow over the edges when subjected to stress.
- The ideal material does not conduct temperature changes or electrical impulses. Thermal and electrical shock can damage the pulp of a tooth.
- The material must have a favorable coefficient of expansion. This is the amount a material expands when heated. If the filling material expands more or less than the tooth structure, then every time you drink coffee or ice water the filling and the tooth change dimensions at different rates. This results in filling margins that leak and may lead to the filling actually popping out.

Silver Amalgam

Silver amalgam is the most commonly used filling material today, and, properly used, a very good material it is. It is unaesthetic, and it too readily conducts temperature and electricity, but otherwise is close to an ideal material. The composition of various brands of silver amalgams varies somewhat, but generally speaking, amalgam is about half silver and half mercury with small amounts of copper, tin, and zinc. Quacks claim that amalgam is poisonous because of the mercury. The claim is untrue, but thousands of people have had their mouths mutilated because of this false claim. (Chapter 20 gives full coverage to this noxious practice.)

To prepare amalgam, a machine blends the ingredients. The mercury dissolves the metallic powders, thus forming a solution. At this point the mass is malleable, but it will soon begin to harden, ultimately forming a strong, solid alloy. The filling is made while the mix is easily manipulated. The filling is carved or shaped as it is beginning to set, and then polished after it is set. You are usually cautioned not to bite down hard on the new filling for a day, until it hardens completely.

Although a carefully conceived and well-made silver-amalgam filling can last indefinitely, barring accident and assuming reasonable home care, failures do occur. Most are caused by poor dentistry, but even good work sometimes fails. Stress placed too soon on a new and still brittle amalgam filling can cause a hairline fracture that sometimes goes undetected for years, until continued stress dislocates a piece of the filling. Occasionally a tooth wall proves too weak to support the filling, and sooner or later the tooth itself cracks at its weak point, necessitating a new restoration. Such a break usually leaves the filling still in place and intact; this shows how strong the filling material can be. Sometimes poor oral hygiene sabotages the dentist's efforts by undermining a filled tooth with new decay.

All these types of failure are quite rare in the case of good restorations. In general, well-made fillings *do not come out.* The failure of *poor* restorations, on the other hand, is virtually inevitable. The notion that well-made silver fillings are impermanent is nonsense. Yet patients have told me that their dentist tried to "sell" them gold inlays to replace amalgam fillings because "silver fillings don't last." Of course, if the inlay work is of the same quality as the amalgam work, the inlays won't last either.

The reasons for the failure of poor amalgam fillings are numerous, but all can be explained by haste and inattention to detail.

It is impossible to give careful attention to all details and complete the operation in a few minutes, as Dr. Poorwork does. It is his calculated inattention to such matters that is responsible for nearly all these failures. How does Dr. Poorwork justify his behavior? A Poorwork we know once said, "I make a filling that will hold the tooth for a few years. Isn't that worth fifty bucks?" We told him that holding a tooth together for a few years is indeed worth fifty bucks, but *only if the work is truthfully represented.* We would have no complaints about Dr. Poorwork if he always represented his work for what it is: substandard and inadequate. But as long as the patient thinks that one dentist's filling is as good as another's, as the American Dental Association leads him to believe, then he tends to select the least expensive dentist and is deprived of a real choice.

Aesthetic Fillings

Although amalgam, properly used, is a fine filling material, it is unsuitable for use in the front of the mouth, where the filling can be seen. For years we used silicate cement or acrylic, but both materials had serious shortcomings. A new type of substance, although still not perfect, is infinitely superior. These new materials are known generically as composites and are essentially plastics combined with other materials. When they are used carefully, they make superb fillings for front teeth, both aesthetically and functionally. Researchers are improving these composite materials all the time, but they are still considered by most authorities to be inferior to amalgam for large back tooth fillings. However, composites may soon improve to the point that we can, with a nostalgic shrug, say good-bye to the old silver-amalgam filling. But not just yet. (Refer to the section on composite inlays later in this chapter.)

Dr. Poorwork's results with composite materials are particularly dismal. As with everything else in dentistry, each step in the preparation of a composite filling must be done with meticulous care, and each step takes time! Composites are difficult to use properly but easy to use sloppily. So Poorwork too often smears in composite materials, usually charging a premium for using the "new cosmetic filling"!

Pins

Dentists often use small pins to help hold very large silver or composite fillings. These pins are typically placed by drilling very small holes into the tooth and then screwing in the pin. Because the tooth is made of breakable material, pins can lead to serious fractures, especially if they are placed too close to the outside of the tooth. If, on the other hand, they are placed far from the outside, they can poke into the nerve, requiring future root canal therapy. With all these problems, we don't like pins to retain fillings. Fortunately, the new bonding techniques allow dentists to add retention without the use of pins. If the filling is so large that bonding won't work, a crown or inlay is indicated.

BONDING

"Bonding" is the general term given to the myriad chemical adhesive techniques developed in the last generation. Bonding techniques involve etching the tooth surface with an acid and then attaching adhesive chemicals to the microscopically rough-etched surface. Bonded composites can repair broken, stained, and discolored teeth and close spaces between front teeth. Veneers on crowns and bridgework can be easily repaired, and large silver fillings can be veneered for aesthetics using these materials.

The bonding technique is also used to lower a child's susceptibility to decay on the chewing surfaces of his permanent back teeth. In this technique, the biting surfaces of the teeth are etched and covered with composite material, called in this case sealants. In our opinion sealants are greatly overused. We feel they should be used only on permanent teeth that have deep grooves prone to decay. Dr. Fraud loves to smear sealants on all of his young patients and often falsely reports them to the insurance carrier as permanent fillings.

Laminates are different: unlike bondings, which are done in the dental chair right on the teeth, laminates are made in the laboratory from impressions taken by the dentist after the teeth are prepared by being ground down a bit in the front. The tooth-colored laminates are then attached to the teeth at a later appointment. Laminates are usually made of porcelain, but they also can be made of composite plastics. They involve greater expense than ordinary bondings but generally provide a more reliable aesthetic result.

Silver-amalgam fillings also can be bonded to the tooth. Early results with this technique are extremely promising, although no long-term studies are available.

Bondings have their downside. Despite the claims of some dentists, bondings are an invasive process, usually requiring some grinding of the teeth. Bondings are *not* a substitute for crowns. Although bondings can be done for aesthetic problems where in the past crowns would have been necessary, when crowns are needed functionally, only crowns will do. Bondings should be used only for aesthetic correction. Over the years some bondings stain and discolor; often they can be polished successfully, but sometimes they have to be redone. They do not stand up well to heavy chewing, and dentists must try to use them where they will not receive sizable chewing impact. Bonding techniques can be used as a temporary measure to replace front teeth, with a replacement tooth bonded to adjacent teeth, but this is not suitable as a permanent restoration. Well-done bondings can last a long time, but for a variety of reasons occasionally must be redone at shorter intervals. Laminates seem to have a better prognosis but haven't been around long enough to have a definitive judgment made. And, as one might expect, bonding procedures in the hands of Dr. Poorwork can be a disaster. We recently saw a young woman with front teeth that had been veneered two years ago. They were a peculiar color and getting somewhat painful. Examination showed that Dr. Poorwork had installed expensive laminates by smushing bonding materials over decay. By this time the teeth were almost rotted away and required major reparative and restorative dentistry.

Despite these reservations, bonding is an immensely helpful technique when used appropriately. Depending on the skill and care of the dentist, and on other factors such as the biting stress on the restored areas, bondings can give superb long-term aesthetic results. Bonding provides an inexpensive and excellent solution to some previously awkward dental problems.

INLAYS

An inlay is a filling that is made outside the mouth and cemented in place in the prepared tooth. The cast-gold inlay is a venerable procedure which, when carefully done, produces excellent results.

It is very strong, having greater edge strength and crushing strength than amalgam. But because it is made outside the mouth from impressions and models of the prepared tooth, it cannot fit as exactly as an amalgam filling, which is formed directly in the tooth itself. The inlay is cemented into the tooth, and any inaccuracies of fit are filled in by cement. However, this cement may wash out over time, leaving a leak in the restoration. This is the major disadvantage of the gold inlay.

A bonded composite inlay made of plastic materials has a superior seal to the gold inlay. It remains to be seen whether the composite inlays will hold up as well over the years. We see gold inlays (and amalgams) that are half a century old and still functioning well. We hope we'll be able to say the same thing in the future about the composite inlays.

Some of our New Age friends seem to think that the older a treatment is the better it is: acupuncture, for example. They will be pleased to know that the method we use for making metal-cast crowns and inlays was used more than four thousand years ago by the Babylonians. It's called the lost-wax method (described in Chapter 12).

The types of fillings we have been discussing are all examples of so-called permanent fillings. Their permanence must not be taken literally, of course; though the good dentist and the patient would like them to last forever, many will not.

So-called temporary fillings, which should be used rarely, are stopgaps intended to be replaced by permanent restorations as soon as possible. Occasionally a tooth requires sedative medication, for example, when pulp-capping or pulpotomy procedures are being performed; in such cases the temporary filling acts as a vehicle for the medication. (Recently developed methods for pulp-capping using adhesive bonding techniques allow a permanent filling to be placed immediately.) Temporary fillings can also be used legitimately to protect a tooth while an inlay is being made for it. Occasionally, furthermore, a dentist finds widespread, serious decay and wants to clean out all decay in the teeth involved at once, before making permanent restorations. These are all good, if very special, reasons for using temporaries.

On the other hand, the *routine* use of temporary fillings is bad dentistry. Routine temporaries are dear to the heart of Dr. Poorwork. One reason for this is that his patients are accustomed to paying a certain fee per visit; the temporary filling increases the number of visits. And since Poorwork rarely takes the time to remove all decay from a tooth, the sedative medication of the temporary filling, much of which is left in the tooth under the to-be-made silver filling, soothes the pulp and delays the inevitable toothache. By the time the toothache does finally occur and the tooth is extracted, the patient will have forgotten that the filling was done relatively recently and won't connect the filling with the extraction.

10. Periodontal Disease

*

Periodontal disease (once called pyorrhea) refers to the inflammation and loss of the gums and the supporting tissues of the teeth, and is the major cause of tooth loss. It is paradoxical that tooth loss is caused more often by trouble with the gums than by trouble with the tooth. The ADA states that *more than half* of the population over the age of eighteen shows signs of the early stage of periodontal disease. Yet the treatment of this disease is often neglected by many dentists who should, and usually do, know better. A special tragedy of periodontal disease is that it frequently causes the loss of perfectly sound, decay-free teeth. "The teeth are fine, but the gums gotta go" has become a cliché because it so often true.

In addition to being a leading cause of tooth loss, periodontal disease also results in pain, mouth odors, an unattractive mouth, and a general sense of not feeling very well. In advanced cases the gums can be swollen, red, and ooze pus, which is continuously swallowed. Periodontal disease is usually characterized by chronic discomfort rather than sharp acute pain, but when the infection around the teeth and under the gums gets beyond the body's ability to control, severe painful swellings (periodontal abscesses) can erupt. Teeth with gum disease are often sensitive to cold and may be quite loose. Many people exhibit these symptoms in spite of going to a dentist routinely, never knowing the relief that proper treatment can afford them until it is too late, and the teeth are lost.

The major cause of periodontal disease is neglect, either by the patient who fails to properly and regularly clean his teeth or by the dentist who ignores the warning signs of disease and performs perfunctory exams and cleanings. The gums, jawbone, and ligaments that connect the teeth to the jawbone are called the periodontal tissues. Disease and destruction of any part of these tissues lead to loosening and eventual loss of the affected teeth. The disease takes a rather predictable course, starting with bleeding gums and advancing to swollen, inflamed, and painful gums, ending with loosening teeth and then tooth loss. Although nearly all people with periodontal disease go through these stages, often they are unaware that they even have the disease until it's too late. That's because the symptoms are slow and almost undetectable, until the destruction is advanced. Of course, these symptoms are not undetectable to the good dentist who examines for bone loss by probing the gums and taking X rays, and carefully checks for inflammation and infection. There are rare instances, however, where the disease suddenly affects an area of the mouth despite careful home care by the patient and competent care by the dentist. In such cases the course of the disease is usually atypical, affecting just one or a few teeth.

MEDIA-GENERATED MYTHS

Madison Avenue has capitalized on the misery of victims of periodontal disease with the dissemination of misleading notions and wholly inaccurate information. "Bad breath," "pink toothbrush," "bleeding, messy gums," an "army marching through your mouth"—these are all advertisers' euphemisms for the common symptoms of periodontal problems. The ads promote particular over-the-counter products as being effective for treating some of these symptoms (at the same time proclaiming that the products also add to the user's sex appeal). The truth is, however, that the *only* way to deal effectively with periodontal disease is with thorough periodontal therapy performed by a capable dentist in conjunction with appropriate home care. Periodontal disease cannot be cured with drugs, toothpaste, mouthwashes, vitamins, or food supplements. It's true that the flavorings in some of these preparations mask the odors for a few minutes while they wash away some of the excess pus, but this is hardly our idea of sex appeal.

Periodontal disease is considered to be the most widespread disease of people over the age of forty. Because of a large increase in the number of gum specialists (periodontists) and the public's hunger for simple solutions, the amount of attention and information concerning the disease has significantly increased. But much of this information is only partially true, and much is misleading. For example, many people still believe that pyorrhea is contagious, inherited, and incurable. All these notions are only partially correct. The germs seemingly involved in periodontal disease are found in most people's mouths; for unknown reasons these germs cause disease in some susceptible people but not in others. Getting gum disease from another person, while possible, has not been confirmed. Although the tendency to develop gum disease may be inherited, this is certainly a minor factor in the development of the disease and can be overcome with proper preventive measures. With few exceptions, periodontal disease is treatable and controllable and does not need to lead to "false teeth."

THE BEST—AND WORST—TREATMENTS

Research into the causes and treatment of periodontal disease is going at a rapid pace. The most currently accepted theory is that susceptible adults who neglect (or whose dentist neglects) to remove all the food that the ever-present mouth bacteria digest suffer from both the end products of that digestion and from the body's attempt to control the bacterial toxins. This immune response can be too intense, leading to resorption of the bone around the tooth and further inflammation. It has also been determined that adolescents and children sometimes suffer from a distinct and rapidly advancing type of periodontal disease called juvenile periodontosis. Advanced adult or juvenile periodontal dis-

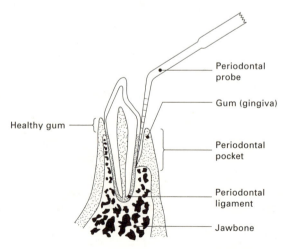

Measuring a Periodontal Pocket

ease are often beyond the competence of the general practitioner and requires the expertise of the specialist.

Effective treatment must begin with an accurate diagnosis, and this requires that the dentist carefully assess the presence and depth of any periodontal defects around the teeth. He is looking specifically for gum that has receded or that has separated from the tooth. This is best accomplished with X rays, and a periodontal probe. The perio probe is calibrated in millimeters. The dentist places it carefully between the tooth and the gum and measures how far it penetrates and if the gums bleed when it is removed. Charting of the pockets is useful to track the progress of the disease. Dr. Poorwork rarely does a probing or charting. If your dentist has never probed your gums, ask why.

The most important and easiest factor to control in periodontal disease is oral hygiene. If there are no food residues in the mouth to feast on, or plaque and tartar to live on, the bacteria responsible for causing perio disease cannot multiply in sufficient numbers to do any harm. Therefore, periodontal therapy is geared toward cleaning the mouth, removing all food residues, plaque, and tartar, and making it easier for the patient to keep the mouth clean. This involves teaching the patient proper oral hygiene methods, and also correcting defective and ill-fitting dental restorations that catch and trap food debris. Treatment begins with thorough scalings (scraping away plaque and tartar) after which, if there has been much bone loss, periodontal surgery may be necessary. After periodontal treatment, any missing teeth can be replaced. And finally the patient will be required to visit both the dentist and periodontist two to six times a year, to appraise the health of the mouth and to do regular cleanings.

Periodontal surgery is sometimes needed to stop the progress of gum disease. Modern surgical approaches vary, but they all share certain steps. The gums are anesthetized and carefully flapped back from the underlying bone, diseased tissue is removed, and the tooth roots are scraped and cleaned. The gum tissue is shortened and then sutured back in place. A dressing, called a periodontal pack, is put over the gums to protect them. Sutures and dressings are removed in about a week.

The surgical procedures, usually done with local anesthetics, are painless. Some discomfort after the surgery is common, and the teeth may be sensitive to hot and cold for a while, but any pain is easily controlled by medication. The idea of periodontal surgery is frightening to many people and can be quite expensive, but it is now a routine part of dentistry and gives excellent results when performed properly.

Periodontal surgery is an area much abused by poorworks, frauds, and quacks. It is too easy and tempting to muck about the gums a bit and report "surgery" on the insurance form; this is sadly true of some poorwork periodontists we know.

Cleanings are an area where Dr. Poorwork cuts corners almost every time. A proper cleaning always requires careful scaling of the teeth using metal instruments. These thin sharp scalers are inserted under the gums and pushed and pulled against the tooth, removing the tartar and smoothing the tooth so that it is more difficult for new tartar to attach itself. For cleanings, some Poorworks only use an ultrasonic cleaning device, or an apparatus that blasts a high-pressure stream of mild abrasive. Then some simply polish the teeth without any scaling at all. The ultrasonic device is excellent for removing heavy tartar, but it is still essential that the dentist or hygienist use hand instruments to meticulously remove any remaining particles of tartar and, most important, smooth and polish the tooth where the tartar was attached. This is painstaking, tedious work; like other dental procedures, it takes time. The abrasive device is useful only for removing stains and has no effect on tartar under the gums. It is therefore useless in treating or preventing periodontal disease since its effect is only cosmetic.

Poorworks also like to use mouthwashes, and many are advocates of the discredited baking soda and peroxide method of cleaning teeth. This method, also called the Keyes technique, is fully explained in Chapter 20, but it is important to note that the baking soda and peroxide method has not been shown to offer any advantages over regular toothpaste in cleaning the teeth or controlling gum disease. This technique does lessen the superficial symptoms, but the disease continues to advance until the patient's teeth are beyond salvation. We call this "supervised neglect." But since Dr. Poorwork is interested in creating more work for himself, such neglect is an added incentive.

The bulk of Dr. Poorwork's dental work is always limited to what his patients will readily accept and pay for at rates that return a healthy profit for the limited amount of time Poorwork invests. Periodontal treatment makes Poorwork unhappy because it takes too much time, time for which his patients are not accustomed to paying. Poorwork is capable of diagnosing periodontal disease and knows that it leads to pain and tooth loss. But his patients are used to a "cleaning": a polishing that takes just a few minutes and a perfunctory scaling called a "gum treatment." Masking the symptoms with peroxide mouthwashes, applications of gentian violet, and, in some cases, even antibiotic prescriptions is far quicker and easier and more in line with the fees Poorwork's patients accept without question. Unfortunately, many patients have never had a thorough cleaning so don't know that they are being shortchanged.

Peroxide can work superficially to reduce inflammation, often convincing the patient that his gum problems are "cured," and all the while the bacteria are continuing to destroy the tooth's support system under the gums. Gentian violet is left over from the days when a dentist would get paid only if he "did something," and the patient was happy only if the doctor "put something on it." This dye has absolutely no effect other than turning the gums purple. But many patients are convinced (and happy to pay for) the purple gum treatment of Dr. Poorwork. You might ask, "Why isn't Dr. Poorwork sued when his patients lose their teeth?" The answer is that Poorwork's patients have been taught that pyorrhea is incurable and that tooth loss is inevitable, and they quietly accept their fate.

There are excellent, honest, reputable periodontists who diagnose accurately and treat properly with superb results. But there are others whose fraudulent diagnoses and treatment plans are matched only by their incompetence. We've seen full-mouth surgery (a major and expensive procedure) performed on patients who had not a trace of periodontal disease. We've seen collusion between general dentists and specialists to defraud patients. In one case the general dentist recommended his patient to the specialist for extensive periodontal treatment; the specialist in turn recommended that the general dentist do extensive crown and bridgework for this patient following completion of the periodontal treatment. Both dentists knew that the patient's teeth could not be saved, yet they took thousands of dollars from her, putting her through annoying treatments that in a short while failed completely.

Finding a good periodontist can be hazardous. Some dentists recommend only their friends and golf partners, which is not a good way to get a recommendation. Checking the local dental school faculty may be worthwhile, but since there are many bad periodontists (as well as good ones) on dental school faculties or associated with teaching hospital clinics, there is still no guarantee. The best recommendation will probably come from a good general dentist, but it never hurts to get a few opinions when major dentistry is needed.

RISK FACTORS

Current research is directed to identifying the risk factors associated with developing periodontal disease. At this time dentists do not have a usable and accurate way to predict who will get gum problems and what will happen to those patients already diagnosed as suffering from gum disease. One of the problems is that we still haven't isolated specific bacteria involved in causing periodontal disease.

It is known that such factors as smoking, oral hygiene, age, diabetes, and the presence of some specific bacteria are useful as predictors, but the patient's own susceptibility and response to the bacteria appear to be at least equally important. There are data suggesting a genetic link, but this has not been scientifically established. Smoking has been shown to have an association with tooth loss; in one study, people with poor oral hygiene lost more teeth if they smoked than if they didn't.

Certain drugs such as cyclosporin A, which is given to organ transplant patients, have been associated with the growth of excessive gum tissue. This can also be caused by antiepileptic drugs such as Dilantin, and by certain drugs used to manage angina and hypertension.

Some companies are marketing microbiological testing kits for use by dentists in diagnosing periodontal disease. None of these tests is accurate enough to be used. They are experimental, and you should not be charged for an experiment. The best way to diagnose periodontal health is still with X rays and mechanical probing of the gums for pockets (manual and electronic probes are equivalent in accuracy). Your dentist should probe for pockets whenever you have an examination, at least once a year.

Considerable research is being done to improve the treatment of periodontal disease with antimicrobial agents. Although advanced gum disease is still treated with a combination of deep cleanings, meticulous home care, and gum surgery, the future holds promise for reducing surgery and substituting treatments based on systemic drugs and topical mouthwashes. The benefits of chlorhexidine mouthwashes have been established; although they don't cure disease they do help control it. Antibiotic-impregnated fibers have shown promise: They look similar to floss and are inserted under the infected gums after scalings are done. But these fibers are difficult to use and are not advised for patients with poor home care. Systemically administered antibiotics have been shown to help resolve periodontal disease, but long-term antibiotic therapy is rarely advisable.

Some dentists are using a prescaling gel to make the removal of tartar easier. The gel contains chemicals to soften the tartar and detergents to wash it away, but a double-blind study found the gel no more effective than a placebo.

The use of Gore-Tex membranes in periodontal surgery to predictably "guide" tissue healing has become popular and continues to expand as new products and applications are produced. This technique, called guided tissue regeneration (GTR), shows particular promise in resolving one of dentistry's most intractable problems, the loss of bone between the roots of molars. Although most research shows GTR to help regrow some bone, the available methods have been evaluated and found not to provide satisfactory results for the most severe bone defects.

Resorbable synthetic material and transplanted bone are also being used to fill in bone defects. The scientific data appear promising for these materials, but they are still not a predictable cure for advanced bone loss. These techniques can be safely undertaken, but you should discuss the rationale, risks, and chances of success with your periodontist and your general dentist (very few general dentists have the training to work with these materials).

In the future, certain growth factors may increase the success of periodontal therapy. Of course, medicines that are capable of helping are also capable of harming, so more research has to be done to detect any side effects before these new drugs are released for the public.

TRENCH MOUTH

Trench mouth got its name because it was widespread in the trenches of World War I. Today it is known as acute necrotizing ulcerative gingivitis (ANUG), a painful infection of the gums that results from very poor oral hygiene. It is seen most commonly among teenagers who have bad hygiene, don't get enough sleep, and have a poor diet, conditions also prevalent in the trenches. ANUG is not periodontal disease, but if left untreated it can lead to periodontal disease.

Although a full-blown case of ANUG can be very painful, its treatment is relatively simple: Clean the mouth, using warm water rinses, good hygiene, and, if needed, medication. Scaling should be done as soon as the tenderness in the gums subsides. For medication we prefer a chlorhexidine mouthwash to systemic antibiotics, but there are times when only antibiotics will bring the acute disease under control.

We've often had patients tell us that their gum problems began with "a case of trench mouth" when they were teenagers, and that is why their teeth were eventually lost. The implication that the ANUG caused the adult periodontal problems results from a series of misconceptions. The first episode of ANUG was a warning of poor oral hygiene, and this continued poor oral hygiene eventually brought on the adult periodontal disease. The habits remained the same, but the diseases are quite different. It's very likely that the patient's first bout of ANUG was improperly treated, perhaps only with an over-the-counter mouthwash, followed by cursory cleanings and no proper instruction in oral health care. The end result, of course, was full-blown periodontal disease.

THE BOTTOM LINE

A good dentist regularly checks the periodontal condition of his patients. X rays and a perio probe are necessities, as are routine scalings and home care instruction. Brushing and flossing are essential, and most over-the-counter mouthwashes and toothpastes are of little value (see Chapter 17). It is not normal for the gums to bleed when they are brushed; bleeding usually means that a scaling is overdue. If your gums bleed frequently, and your dentist treats you with a perfunctory "cleaning" and mouthwashes, it may be time to look for another dentist.

Periodontal disease is controllable. The bone that has been lost will never regrow, but with proper treatment, no further bone loss need occur. Dramatic successes have been achieved even in what seemed to be nearly hopeless cases. The experience of modern practice and scientific studies has convinced us that, if preventive care is started early enough by both the dentist and the patient, almost no one need lose his teeth because of periodontal disease.

11. Root Canal

*

The science of root canal therapy has become very sophisticated since the days of using extremely caustic and dangerous chemicals, such as arsenic, to "kill" the nerve. Today root canal procedures are so effective that there is hardly ever any reason to extract a tooth because of infection or inflammation of the pulp, or because of pain. And in the great majority of cases, the procedure, if properly done, *is painless*. Even with this impressive record, many people still harbor the ancient belief that an abscessed tooth must be extracted. Contributing to misinformation is Dr. Poorwork, who, unwilling to take the time needed for careful root canal treatment, may either extract salvageable teeth or botch the root canal therapy. We have seen many people terrified of root canal because they have heard of or directly experienced Dr. Poorwork's version of root canal, with the consequent extreme pain and, too often, loss of the tooth anyway.

So what *is* root canal therapy? A healthy tooth is hollow, and the hollow space (the root canal) is filled with living tissue called the pulp, comprised of nerves, blood vessels, and connective tissue. The pulp is often called the "nerve." Although the pulp is not actually a nerve, it is an extremely sensitive tissue: Anything that touches or irritates the pulp also triggers the nerve fibers in the pulp to fire. Often the result is intense pain. Root canal therapy is the removal of the infected pulp and the cleaning and widening and filling of the root canal.

REVERSIBLE AND IRREVERSIBLE PULPITIS

Many things can irritate the pulp: decay, biting too hard, very hot or cold food or drink, a very deep filling, dental work on the tooth for any reason, abnormal habits such as using teeth to open bottles, trauma, or serious periodontal problems that allow bacteria to penetrate near the tip of the root. But an irritated pulp doesn't always require root canal therapy. There are two kinds of pulp inflammation, reversible and irreversible; the dentist must determine which one of these conditions the patient has. A reversible pulpitis (also called hyperemia) can be treated with conservative therapies such as eating softer foods or slightly adjusting the bite on the tooth. If the tooth is decayed, removing the decay and putting in a proper filling usually solve the problem. But if the inflammation is irreversible, the only sensible solution is root canal therapy; the only alternative treatment is the unsatisfactory one of extracting the tooth.

Tooth decay is the most common cause of pulpitis. Cavities, if untreated, relentlessly continue their course toward the pulp. The progress may be fast or slow, depending on individual susceptibility and other factors, but, *always,* as the decay advances and the pulp retreats from it, the decay wins the race and the tooth begins to show symptoms. Usually sensitivity to sweets is an early symptom, but later the tooth becomes dreadfully sensitive to temperature and pressure. The sensitivity occurs because the pulp swells, just as other inflamed tissues would, but there is no room for swelling within the hard, rocklike tooth walls of the root canal. This pressure builds up quickly, and soon the owner of the tooth experiences considerable pain.

The inflammatory process proceeds until there is sufficient pressure inside the tooth to force material out from the tiny opening at the tip of the root, the apex, and into the surrounding bone, causing destruction of the bone along with extreme pain. This bone destruction can usually be detected on an X ray as a darkened area around the tip of the root and is a sure sign of an irreversible pulpitis. We call this area an abscess. The bacteria that exit the apex can cause generalized swelling of the gum and cheek surrounding the area of infection and can lead to a severe infection called a cellulitis. The classic image of a person with a handkerchief wrapped around a swollen face is often portrayed as comical—but there is nothing funny about the possible serious consequences of this type of major infection. Paradoxically, pain decreases when the swelling occurs; as the pus escapes into the soft tissues causing the swelling, the pressure inside the tooth's root canal and on the surrounding bone is relieved. However, a cellulitis is serious, can be fatal, and must be treated promptly.

A cellulitis can almost always be treated successfully with root canal therapy and antibiotics. But long-standing tooth infections are sometimes impossible to clear up without surgically opening the bone and cleaning out the infection. This process is called an apicoectomy and involves the surgical removal of the tip of the root.

If you examine the skulls of ancient men at the Museum of Natural History you will see that many of the displayed jaws have holes in them. Many of these ancients, born before the days of root canal, died of these jaw abscesses. As history proceeded, Man learned to extract these painful teeth: pulling the tooth established a pathway for the drainage and resolution of the infection. Often the tissue formed by the body defense system around the apex of the root would come out with the extracted tooth. This tissue, looking somewhat like a worm, gave rise to the ancient theory that toothache was caused by a worm.

ROOT CANAL THERAPY

Root canal therapy consists of several steps and usually requires at least two visits to the dentist. He first drills a small hole in the top of the infected tooth. The pulp is removed, and medication is placed and sealed into the tooth with a temporary filling. At the next appointment the temporary filling and medication are removed, X rays are taken to determine exactly how long the roots are, and, if the infection is gone, the dentist fills the roots of the tooth with a special material, usually made with gutta percha. (See Chapter 11 for a review of other root canal filling materials.)

In common with all other aspects of dentistry, endodontics (meaning inside the tooth) can be done poorly, carelessly, and with unproven filling materials. Many people believe that root-canal-treated teeth turn black. This is rare and usually reflects a hastily done procedure in which some of the pulp tissue was left in the tooth; this, in time, discolors the remaining tooth structure. Sometimes bleaching can correct this; at other times a crown, veneer, or bonding can be done for cosmetic reasons.

Dr. Poorwork doesn't often try to save teeth, but when he does, his methods are determined by the amount of time he is willing to spend. Often the infected tooth is opened and a chemical, such as silver nitrate or formaldehyde, is used to "kill" the nerve. This is far

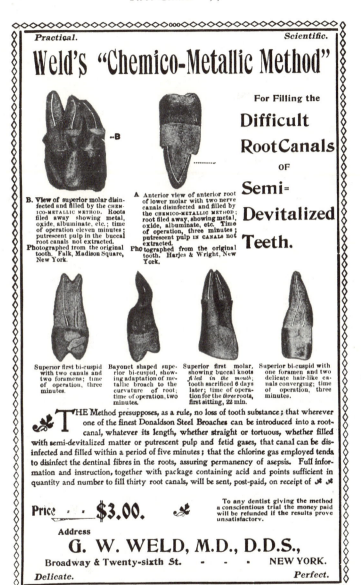

Weld's Chemico-Metallic Method. An 1897 ad for a "five minute" root canal therapy. The dentist/physician who marketed this product did not list the active ingredient nor did he mention any side effects. This was typical of ads before the first Food and Drug Law in 1906. (Illustration from *Items of Interest,* A Monthly Magazine of Dental Art, Science and Literature, September 1897.)

easier than meticulously removing the pulp tissue. Dr. Poorwork often follows this chemical treatment with a halfhearted root canal filling that doesn't completely fill the root. At times even this perfunctory treatment meets with success because of the body's amazing ability to heal itself.

Some quacks compound incompetence with the preposterous claim that all teeth that have already been saved with root canal therapy must be extracted. They claim that this can cure problems throughout the body and lessen the symptoms of diseases as diverse as arthritis and Parkinson's disease. Of course this is nonsense, but the replacement of the extracted teeth can be very profitable. (See Chapter 20.)

Pulpitis and associated pain are not the only reasons for doing root canal therapy. Sometimes the pulp degenerates over a period of time without symptoms, the tooth becoming what dentists call "nonvital." This condition, if untreated, can lead to cyst formation, jaw weakening, and painful, acute, infectious flare-ups. It is diagnosable by X rays and must be treated by root canal therapy.

Sometimes endodontic treatment is necessary on a structurally weakened tooth so that a post can be made to support a crown. A post is a metal rod cemented into the prepared root canal that helps hold the crown to a weak tooth. Posts should be fitted and cemented into place. Posts that are screwed into root canals are popular, but they tend to fracture the root, causing loss of the tooth; we prefer the fitted and cemented posts.

At times weak teeth, even roots, can be preserved with root canal and used to support attachments for removable dentures. When used in this way, the denture is called an overdenture because it goes over the root-canal-treated roots that have received special types of attachments to help hold the denture in place.

As you can see, root canal therapy is a very useful, safe, and effective means of saving teeth that would otherwise need to be extracted. Remember: Root canal—if done properly—is almost always *painless,* and here, as in every aspect of dental care, taking sufficient time to do it right is the essential element.

12. Crowns

*

Crowns are among the most expensive dental procedures and yet most people have very little understanding of what they really are, when they should be used, and what steps are necessary to achieve an excellent result.

Anatomically, a tooth is divided into crown and root, the crown being that part of the tooth visible above the gums. In the dental restorative sense a crown is an artificial replacement that restores the natural crown of the tooth. A crown is made when the tooth's natural crown is so badly damaged that a filling will not suffice, or when the tooth is needed as an anchor tooth for a bridge (see Chapter 14), or, occasionally, for cosmetic reasons.

A restoration that covers the whole visible tooth is called a full crown. Crowns differ in the purpose for which they are intended and in the material used. They can be made of gold, base metal, porcelain fused to the metal, metal veneered with plastic, stainless steel (used for temporary repairs to back teeth), acrylic plastic (used for temporary repairs to front teeth), and all-porcelain (also called jackets if placed on the front teeth). But the criteria for a proper crown are the same for all, except the temporary crowns that need not be as exact.

A properly made crown is an excellent, long-lasting restoration. Even severely decayed teeth, as long as they are surrounded by healthy gums, can be salvaged with a crown. Sometimes even half a tooth can be saved by removing the damaged half and restoring the sound remnant.

Teeth that have been decayed down to the gum line are salvageable with root canal therapy and a post restoration, in which a metal post is cemented in a prepared and widened root canal, giving additional support to the crown. Screw posts are also used, where a post is actually screwed into the canal, but this frequently damages the tooth. A prefabricated post cemented into a prepared root canal does not tend to split the root as does a screw post and is therefore a safer and preferred technique.

Crowns have a number of uses besides repairing otherwise hopeless teeth. Full crowns are the best anchors for fixed bridges and for joining loose teeth together (called splinting). In many types of removable partial dentures, crowns placed on the anchor teeth allow the partial to be made without any visible clasps. But in any elaborate fixed bridge, splint, or oral rehabilitation, the restoration can be no better than the quality of the individual crowns involved. Crowns are also used for strictly cosmetic purposes and are often called by the vernacular term "caps."

In order to construct a crown, enough of the existing tooth must be removed to allow an adequate thickness of the crown material. Usually the dentist uses a high-speed drill to remove tooth structure from the entire visible surface of the tooth. There are a number of different theories about what shape the remainder of the tooth should have, but what is truly important is not the shape but how carefully and accurately the dentist produces the shape. The grinding tapers the tooth so that the crown can slide over it.

After the preparation of the tooth by grinding is complete, the dentist takes an impression of the tooth so that a model of it can be made in the laboratory. There are many different ways of taking an impression. One of the oldest and best ways (and our favorite) is to use a cylinder of copper and fill it with a heat-sensitive material called dental compound. The heated compound is pressed over the tooth, cooled, and removed. Other methods use resilient impression materials. Any method can give a satisfactory result if the dentist takes the time to use it correctly. The dentist will also make a temporary crown that will protect the tooth while the lab is making the final crown.

Other impressions will be needed to establish the relationship to the other teeth in the mouth, showing how wide and how tall the crown must be. If the crown is to be made of metal or contain a metal substructure (as in a porcelain-over-gold crown), the lost-wax technique is used. In this method, invented by the ancient Babylonians, a wax form, made on the model, is placed in a special type of plaster of paris. The wax is melted, leaving a void in the plaster, and then molten metal, usually gold, is forced into the void. This produces an exact replica of the wax form. The replica is called a casting and is remarkably precise.

At a subsequent visit, the dentist tries the crown on to see how it fits. This fitting visit is crucial. The crown is seated on the prepared tooth and painstakingly examined for contact with the adjacent teeth, for bite, and, most important, for the fit at the crown margin (where the crown meets the tooth). This margin is a critical part of the restoration; there must be no sticking out of the margin or opening under the crown. X rays are necessary to verify the exact fit.

FAULTY CROWN MARGINS

Faulty crown margins lead to many problems. If the crown doesn't go all the way to where the dentist ground the tooth down, it's called a short margin, and this leaves some of the tooth uncovered and unprotected. If the margin is too long, it will stick out into the gums and produce periodontal damage. Long margins also chronically irritate the gum tissues and can accelerate bone loss in the area, much like a large piece of tartar. If there is a gap between tooth and crown (open margin), food will be trapped and the tooth is likely to decay.

A faulty margin must be corrected. Sometimes the dentist can trim and closely adapt a margin on the model. (Having a metal model, such as the one a dentist gets with a copper band impression, makes this easier. This is one reason some dentists prefer that impression method). If the margin can't be corrected this way, impressions must be retaken and a new crown made. Once the margins are satisfactorily fitted and trimmed and all other necessary adjustments are made, the crown may be cemented or it may be returned to the lab for more cosmetic alterations. The cosmetics are the easy part; getting the crown to fit is the difficult and essential aspect of doing this procedure.

CEMENTATION

Cementation also requires care. Today dentists have many different types of cement. Because the crown fits so accurately, the cement must be capable of achieving a very thin film thickness while setting very hard. The role of cement is mainly to provide a seal. The poorer the fit of the crown, the more cement will be needed; the greater the thickness of cement, the greater the risk that the ce-

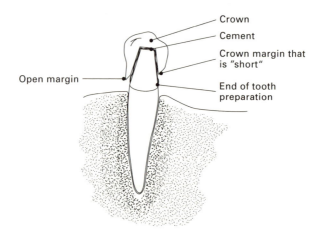

Improperly Fitted Crown

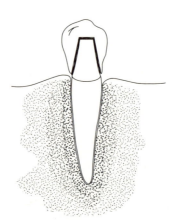

Properly Fitted Crown

ment will eventually dissolve out from under the crown, leading to failure. Good seal can be achieved with a very close adaptation of the margins of the crown to the tooth, coupled with a nearly microscopic thickness of cement.

Don't be upset if your dentist or his assistant refers to a list of instructions before or during cementing a crown. There are now so many cements (the same holds for bonding materials) with so many changes that the dentist cannot keep all these instructions in his head. Some manufacturers of dental cements have small sets of cards designed to be displayed out of the patient's sight so as not to embarrass the dentist when he needs to refer to them. This "cookbook" method of cementation is part of modern dentistry.

Cast-metal crowns are a mainstay of restorative dentistry. Gold has always been the primary metal used, but because of gold's cost other metals, particularly steel alloys, are now more popular. Many dentists, ourselves included, feel that gold alloys are superior and well worth the extra cost, but this point is arguable. Pure gold is too soft for restorative purposes, so the gold is alloyed with other metals, such as copper, silver, platinum and palladium, depending on what properties are desired.

Most people object to metal crowns on aesthetic grounds. To solve this problem, plastic veneers have been attached over gold crowns. But today dentists can produce extremely beautiful crowns from porcelain fused to metal or solid porcelain crowns.

JACKETS (PORCELAIN CROWNS)

Solid porcelain crowns on front teeth have been done successfully for years. Also known as jackets, these porcelain crowns have no metal substructure. Although porcelain is a fairly strong material, it is not as strong as metal and is susceptible to fracture. Nor can it be joined to other crowns with solder joints as can metal restorations. This makes all-porcelain crowns unusable as anchor teeth for fixed bridges. Recent advances in laboratory techniques are producing solid porcelain crowns of great beauty for both front and back teeth, but more time is needed to see if they can hold up to the chewing requirements of the back teeth.

Porcelain crowns also don't have as accurate a marginal fit as do metal crowns, and they're even more difficult to cement, but when used judiciously excellent long-term results have been achieved. As technology improves we expect to see other materials used.

CROWN MAINTENANCE

Crowns often exhibit gum-line discoloration; this is particularly common with porcelain jacket crowns and may be unavoidable, especially if the jacket was made when the patient was much younger. Some recession of the gums as one ages is quite normal, and this may disclose a margin previously covered by the gum. Dentists try to plan for this by placing the margins far enough under the gum, but this is not always possible, especially with young healthy gums. If the margin is truly unsightly, a new jacket may be needed.

Crowning a tooth doesn't guarantee that the tooth will be immune to other problems, although careful maintenance minimizes the risks. Routine examinations are necessary to check on any gum breakdown or marginal decay, and continuing periodontal care is essential. Occasionally we are called upon to remove periodontally diseased teeth with perfectly beautiful crowns. Such a chore is always disheartening.

In short, crown maintenance is the same as tooth maintenance—brush and floss. And don't worry that if you floss around the crown you may pull it off. It is cemented in place.

WHAT TO WATCH OUT FOR

Dr. Poorwork and Dr. Quack also like to try their hands at "cap work" now and then. Dr. Poorwork here again cuts as many corners as possible to produce a quickie crown, minimizing the overhead and maximizing the profit. Poorwork patients show up with open margins, decay left under the crowns, bulging contours, and poor bite. A Poorwork crown can often be detected because the gums around it are discolored, red, swollen, and oozing due to the constant irritation of poorly adapted margins. Occasionally we see a patient with an acrylic crown that was filled with a self-curing plastic and sold to the patient as a porcelain crown. Such a crown is used by good dentists only as a temporary crown while the permanent one is being made; it cannot possibly have properly adapted margins.

Dr. Quack sells unnecessary crowns by telling patients that they're allergic to whatever materials are in their mouths. So crowns that were thought to be perfectly okay turn out to be causing headaches, while the silver fillings are exposed as a poisonous brew causing immune system breakdowns. Of course, Dr. Quack uses weird diagnostic techniques to back up the claims of peril. Crystals, electric devices of every description, reflexology, and sheer chutzpah allow Dr. Quack to persuade many a patient to have unnecessary—and expensive—crowns. (See Chapter 20.)

Dr. Poorwork never spends the time to ensure the meticulous accuracy that enables a good crown to last. A well-made and well-fitted crown in a well-maintained mouth can last a lifetime. But the ubiquity of Dr. Poorwork in dentistry is demonstrated by the fact that insurance companies don't expect crowns to last and will pay for a new crown in three or five years, depending on the coverage. This again illustrates the folly of going to the lowest bidder. In managed care fee-for-service plans, Dr. Poorwork makes a crown quickly and cheaply and is able to make a profit on the low managed care fee. (The poorer the service, the greater the reward.) His crowns might be expected to last three or five years. On the other hand, Dr. Goodwork, who spends three times as long to make a crown, cannot make a profit on the managed care fee. But his crown might last forty years or longer. So because the fee structure encourages Poorwork crowns, the insurer will have to pay again and again for new crowns, and then, as the teeth fail because of the faulty restorations, the insurer will pay for extractions and bridgework, and eventually dentures, all of this avoidable if quality assurance and sufficient fees were part of the program so a good crown could have been made to begin with.

The above holds true for fee-for-service plans. In the increasingly popular "capitation" plans, crowns simply will not be made, because they will cost the dentist more to make than the maximum annual allowance for a patient. (Chapter 21 provides greater detail on this situation.)

13. Oral Surgery and Extractions

✳

All dentists are trained in exodontia, the removal of teeth, but most difficult extractions and surgical procedures beyond the abilities and training of general practitioners are performed by oral surgeons, the second largest group of dental specialists. Routine extractions can normally be performed by the general dentist but many dentists, to avoid the bother and complications associated with extractions, prefer to refer them to an oral surgeon.

Although extractions make up most of the volume of an oral surgeon's practice, oral surgeons are trained for far more difficult procedures such as treating jaw fractures, tumors, salivary gland diseases, and bone irregularities, as well as diagnosing all kinds of oral pathology. Many oral surgeons are also board certified in administering general anesthesia.

An extraction is ordinarily a relatively simple affair, particularly when compared to the work required to repair a badly damaged tooth. The typical extraction, including anesthesia and assuming careful, cautious workmanship, may take five or ten minutes at most. It is a quick and easy job that hardly taxes the skill or stamina of an experienced dentist. Yet the major part of an oral surgeon's income derives from extractions, most of which can be avoided if the patient experiences good dentistry.

Many of the tens of thousands of wisdom tooth extractions are considered functionally unnecessary. There are specific criteria for removing third molars. Just as not everyone has to have his tonsils removed, so too can many people keep their wisdom teeth. Wisdom teeth should be extracted if they are causing prolonged pain, forming cysts, causing problems by pushing into other teeth, or leading to gum infections. If none of these conditions are met, then they should be left alone. Dentists often exaggerate the dangers posed by third molars. Studies have shown that only 6 percent of wisdom teeth are diseased, and less than 1 percent cause damage to the roots of adjacent teeth. Unnecessary extractions account for a vast amount of dental expenditure, particularly when one adds the additional charges for general IV anesthesia into the formula.

UNNECESSARY EXTRACTION

Oral surgeons, like other specialists, often find themselves in the difficult position of seeing a patient for a procedure that has been recommended by the general dentist but that the patient does not need. Usually the surgeon extracts a tooth, even though he realizes that the tooth should actually be saved. But if he tells the patient the truth, the referring dentist may never send him another patient, hurting the surgeon economically. And the oral surgeon could also be accused of violating the ADA's code of ethics for explaining to the patient how he has been improperly treated.

Most teeth that are extracted could have been saved by modern dental treatment. Of course the oral surgeon knows this, but will he try to talk the patient out of having the tooth pulled? It's an interesting ethical question. Will the oral surgeon take the time to properly diagnose and then completely explain how the tooth could be saved with root canal work, followed by a crown, none of which he does or gets paid for? Or will the oral surgeon shrug his shoulders, extract the tooth, and collect his fee?

The profession of oral surgery is beset by the paradox that people who are highly trained and skilled spend most of their time doing extractions, which require very little of their skills and which they rarely prescribe themselves because the extraction often should not even be performed. Predictably, most oral surgeons have come to terms with this problem without disturbing their moral equilibrium. But the modern, progressive, and responsible surgeon is paying more attention to the doctrine of "informed consent," making an effort to instruct patients that there are alternatives to taking a tooth out.

We hope to see the day when the economics of dentistry are changed to provide incentives to do the best for our patients. In that utopian future we will expect oral surgeons to spend most of their time performing the advanced and necessary surgical procedures they are trained to do, rather than simple extractions which, too often, should not even be done.

THE CONSEQUENCES OF LOSING TEETH

Patients are forever telling us that the extraction of one of their teeth was so difficult that "the dentist was sweating." To explain this, the patient may have been told that he had "very long roots." It seems never to have occurred to these people that, in so many cases, a tooth that is *so sturdy that the dentist had difficulty in removing it* should never have been extracted in the first place! Although the percentage of Americans who lose all their teeth is declining, it is still far too high. One of the major themes of this book is that most teeth should not be extracted. Yet it is also true that not every extraction is evidence of bad dentistry.

Pain and infection are the two major reasons for tooth extraction, yet most teeth exhibiting these serious symptoms can be saved with root canal therapy, periodontal procedures, and antibiotics. In dentistry, pain and infection are properly treated by removing the cause—decay, nerve inflammation, or gum infection—*but not by extraction.*

Even in cases of severe decay, root canal therapy and a post, core, and crown can usually restore the tooth. Sometimes the cost of such work is not worth the risk of the tooth later failing, but if a tooth is very necessary to the patient's health, the good dentist will go to heroic lengths to save it. On the other hand, the dentist should hesitate to do elaborate work on a tooth of little importance.

There are legitimate reasons for removing teeth. Some teeth are so badly decayed they can't be saved. Split or fractured teeth are often impossible to save. The saddest cases are teeth in excellent condition that have lost their supporting bone because of periodontal disease. Here again, there is little that can be done to save them.

If you're looking for a dentist, be wary of the general practitioner who has built a reputation on the basis of his "painless extractions." Remember, the extraction of a routine tooth is probably the easiest job in dentistry. The good general dentist, being in the business of *saving* teeth, is rarely called upon to extract a tooth. So steer clear of the neighborhood dentist who is "so good at extractions" and go to the one who so seldom finds them necessary that most of his patients aren't quite sure whether he pulls teeth well or not.

After losing a tooth, what are the consequences? Usually the answer is replacement with a bridge (see Chapter 14). Many people do not understand why a tooth, especially a back tooth that can't be seen, needs to be replaced. Patients almost always notice the loss of a tooth while chewing, but there are other considerations. The teeth are stabilized in their position by the neighboring teeth surrounding them. When a tooth is lost the adjacent teeth usually start to shift, and this tilting can lead to cleaning and chewing problems that will affect the health of other teeth. As the spaces and chewing pressures on the remaining teeth change, the patient encounters difficulty eating with and cleaning the remaining teeth. Often periodontal disease starts around the tilted teeth because they are trapping food; this can also lead to an increase in decay. The forces generated by biting become unbalanced so that additional stresses are placed on certain teeth. These pressures can damage the jawbone and the gums and lead to periodontal disease.

These dire consequences don't occur in every patient who is missing a back tooth. There are people who have had teeth extracted without replacing them and have suffered relatively little dental damage over several years. Unusually favorable conditions in their mouths provide stability for the remaining teeth and prevent excessive drift. They often find that when they are older and less physically able to clean meticulously the slight shifting is enough to adversely affect their oral hygiene and oral health. For most people an unreplaced extracted tooth results in a serious and potentially crippling dental future.

Some good advice: Except in special cases as those mentioned above, do everything possible to keep your teeth. Even severely broken-down teeth can usually be saved.

14. Replacing Missing Teeth: Bridgework, Dentures, and Implants

*

False teeth go back to ancient times. Artificial teeth have been found in Egyptian tombs, and a skull in an Etruscan tomb dating back to 500 B.C. contained a bridge of ox teeth held together with gold rings. (We wonder if the craftsmen of antiquity promised their customers that their dentures would enhance sex appeal or cure bad breath?)

The branch and specialty of modern dentistry that deals with the replacement of missing teeth and the fabrication of bridges and dentures is known as prosthodontics. To many laypeople and, also, many dentists, the importance of prosthetic dentistry reflects an unhealthy attitude. The stress should always be on preventive and restorative work, which, when properly done, limits prosthetics to congenital situations and accident cases. But it is obvious that anything so nearly ideal is far into the future. We will continue to need false teeth as long as dentistry continues to fail in its first mission, saving teeth.

FULL DENTURES

The toothless patient embodies the ultimate failure of dentistry and is the most difficult to treat satisfactorily. When a patient has lost all of his upper or lower teeth, and implants are not considered an option, a removable full denture is the treatment of last resort. Upper full dentures can be quite comfortable and functional, but lower full dentures are rarely completely satisfactory and often are nightmares. Although the number of Americans who have lost all their teeth is decreasing, far too many people still believe that dentures are an inevitable part of the aging process and that all their dental problems will end when they have no more teeth. Nothing is farther from the truth. Patients with dentures lose a great deal of chewing efficiency and a considerable amount of taste sensation. Full dentures need to be repaired and periodically checked for wear and tear. The plastic denture doesn't change, but as time goes by the tissues under the denture do change, and this leads to loosening of the dentures, sore spots, and potentially dangerous chronic irritations that may be a factor in oral cancer. The gums and jawbones, even without teeth, can develop cysts, tumors, and infections. And so patients with dentures should be regularly examined, usually once a year.

Constructing a denture requires a high degree of skill and experience. Some lab technicians have tried to get legislation passed allowing them to market dentures directly to the public. We recommend caution before committing your health to a nonprofessional. Dr. Poorwork loves dentures because they are lucrative and he can use techniques to make dentures quickly, easily, and cheaply. Of course dentures made this way are not likely to be the best quality, but at least Dr. Poorwork can recognize and diagnose cancers and other oral diseases, which nonprofessional denturists are not trained to do.

Today full-denture patients who have a number of nonsalvageable teeth and for whom implants are not practical usually are treated with what is known as an immediate denture, which is inserted immediately after the teeth are extracted. This helps the tissues to heal properly and allows the patient to avoid walking around without teeth. An immediate denture usually has to be relined after the gum tissues have healed, to adapt to the new shape of the healed tissues. Except for this disadvantage, the immediate denture is a great improvement over the old technique of extracting teeth and then waiting some six weeks for the tissues to heal before taking impressions.

The first step in the treatment of a toothless person is a complete examination, including full-mouth X rays, to check for disease and rule out any jaw conditions that would complicate the denture-making process. Once the dentist is satisfied that the patient is healthy and the jaws in condition to support the denture, impressions can be taken. There are many impression-taking techniques, each with its adherents. Each can probably provide good results, if enough time and care are taken to use the technique properly.

Impressions and measurements of jaw relationships are given

to the technician, who constructs a working model of the jaws using a device that mimics the hinge movements of the jaws. He makes a "try-in" denture, which is usually made of wax, shellac, and the same artificial teeth that will be used in the final denture. This is "tried in," and changes are made as necessary. Once the dentist and patient are satisfied with the bite and appearance of this "try-in" in the patient's mouth, the denture can be completed.

In the case of an immediate denture, the remaining teeth are extracted and the denture inserted at the same visit. Some initial adjustments can be made at this time. The first day is the most challenging. There is often the postoperative pain of the multiple extractions combined with the difficulty of adjusting to a radically new mouth environment. As the days go by, the dentist adjusts the denture as necessary, and the patient comes to learn to handle the denture just as millions of patients have done over history. But time and patience are required.

Perhaps the most common cause of denture problems is unrealistic patient expectations, Patients should be taught exactly what to expect from the completed denture. They should be cautioned that the denture is not bolted into place but merely rests on the tissues; certain movements of the mouth will dislodge the denture, while other movements will tend to keep the denture in place. They must learn to focus on the stabilizing movements while avoiding the dislodging ones. They should also be taught that, while the adjustment period might be difficult and even painful, millions of people have succeeded in learning to handle their dentures, and so will they if they try.

DENTURE COMPLAINTS

There are a number of over-the-counter preparations designed to relieve discomfort caused by dentures. The ointments and liquids to be put on denture sores contain a local anesthetic that indeed relieves the pain. But as a rule, such pain is caused by a bad fit in some area of the denture; unless this situation is corrected, the pain always returns as soon as the anesthetic wears off. Denture sores should be taken to the dentist, who generally has little difficulty correcting whatever it is that causes them. Anesthetic preparations should be used only under his supervision. People who use painkilling ointments, except on the dentist's advice, may perpetuate an irritation of the gums, with serious, even lethal consequences, since these ointments may mask a chronic irritation that could become malignant.

Denture adhesives are among the most widely used over-the-counter products. For years dentists were taught that these adhesives were rarely needed for well-fitting dentures, that they were unsanitary, and that they could damage the patient's tissues. Despite this, the wide use of these adhesives indicated their favorable public acceptance. Recent large-scale studies have confirmed the public's wisdom. Denture adhesives are harmless and can be of great help, especially in retaining a lower denture. However, it takes more time to clean a denture that uses adhesive.

PARTIAL DENTURES

Partial dentures are usually recognized by the wire clasps (disparagingly called "clips") that retain them in a patient's mouth. Because a partial denture replaces only some of the teeth, the remaining teeth can be used to hold the denture securely in the mouth. Partial dentures are usually much more comfortable and functional than full dentures, and they can be constructed with more aesthetic techniques that eliminate or hide the clasps.

The removable partial denture is Dr. Poorwork's favorite restoration. It is easy, quick, and profitable. Because there are still teeth in the patient's mouth, impressions and the bite registration are easy to achieve. Because of the peculiar economic incentives of dentistry, Dr. Poorwork often extracts a salvageable tooth and replaces it with a poorly made partial denture that damages the teeth it clasps on to, necessitating future work. This can be called obsolescence by design.

OVERDENTURES

Sometimes a patient has a few teeth that are not strong enough to support crowns but still can be useful. By doing root canal therapy, lowering the teeth by cutting them off at the gum line, and placing a denture over them, they can help retain the denture. Dentists may place tiny magnets in them, or a number of very small snap-on attachments, that can securely hold the denture. Lessening the leverage on these overdenture teeth prolongs their life and provides the patient with additional support for a denture.

RELINES

The mouth continues to change even after all the teeth have been extracted. After a while a denture needs to be relined, that is, refit to adapt to the changing tissues. The average denture needs to be relined once every five years or so, but some people seem to be able to wear the same denture for decades without developing problems while others find their dentures getting loose every other year.

If the reline is done in the office, the inside of the old denture is roughened up and new self-hardening acrylic plastic is placed in the denture, which is then placed in the patient's mouth. The self-curing acrylic smells and tastes bad and feels as if it is burning the tissue (though it isn't). After the impression is taken, the patient should rinse out several times. If the reline is made in the laboratory, impressions must be taken by the dentist, the denture sent to the lab, then returned, inserted, and adjusted. One disadvantage is that the patient is without the denture for a day or more; some patients have additional dentures made for such emergencies. It takes much more of the dentist's time to do the reline in the office, but it is more convenient for the patient.

Sometimes the tissues are raw and inflamed, often because of an ill-fitting denture. In such cases the dentist can use a temporary reline material in the denture that stays soft and resilient for a long period of time and can be replaced several times until the gums are healthy enough to tolerate the hard plastic reline material. Soft reline materials require more meticulous cleaning and frequent dental checkups.

Remember, a reline is almost like getting a new denture and often requires a number of adjustment appointments.

TAKING CARE OF DENTURES

There are many good commercial denture cleaners, but plain mild soap and water can clean them just as well. Dentures can be soaked overnight in a dilute mixture of white vinegar and water, or one part bleach added to ten parts water. Don't use harsh cleaners such as Comet or Ajax on your dentures. Clean dentures often, preferably after each meal. Small denture brushes are good and can reach inside the denture to remove any food debris. Opinion varies on whether to wear dentures while sleeping. We think as long as the patient is comfortable, wearing the denture at night is perfectly all right. But if the denture is removed at night, it should be put into water or the white vinegar solution. If the denture dries out it can distort and become brittle.

Over the years we've seen many patients who lose or break their dentures. We therefore now recommend that all denture patients have an extra, emergency set of dentures.

FIXED BRIDGES

The fixed partial denture (fixed bridge) is a mainstay of high-quality restorative dentistry and, when feasible, is the preferred way of replacing missing teeth. A properly made fixed bridge is comfortable and convenient, lasts a very long time, and needs little in the way of special hygiene. But successful fixed bridgework requires strong support (abutment) teeth and enough of them to support the span of teeth being replaced; the longer the span, the more abutments needed.

A fixed bridge is convenient, comfortable, and long-lasting. A fixed bridge is called a permanent restoration in that the anchors are cemented in place. Because a fixed bridge evenly distributes the considerable forces of chewing, it is far stronger than a removable partial denture and allows more efficient chewing. If your dentist properly plans and executes a fixed bridge and you take good care of it, you can expect many trouble-free years of use. We've seen many bridges that have been functioning perfectly for over twenty-five years, and thirty- and forty-year-old fixed bridges are not uncommon.

In fixed bridgework, even more than in other areas of dentistry, high levels of skill and meticulous attention to detail are critical to achieving a successful result. Because of this, fixed bridgework is quite expensive to the patient. Yet, because of high laboratory costs and chair time, it does not necessarily return a high profit to the dentist. Removable bridges cost the patient far less and are usually more profitable to the dentist.

The most common type of fixed bridge has a crown at each end with one or two false teeth soldered in between. If there aren't anchor teeth present at each side of a missing tooth, a cantilever bridge with several anchor teeth on only one side and a false tooth hanging off the other side can be constructed. Such a bridge is theoretically unsound because of the enormous leverage exerted on the anchor teeth. Although a cantilever bridge is not considered ideal, it can be used if the anchor teeth are very strong. Dr. Poorwork often uses only one unsuitable anchor tooth to hold a false tooth. This is almost always bound to fail.

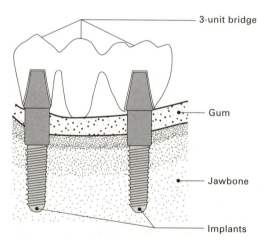

3-unit bridge

Gum

Jawbone

Implants

Two Threaded Implants Supporting a 3-Unit Fixed Bridge

Constructing a fixed bridge is very similar to making a crown, but on a larger scale. In Chapter 12 we described the steps necessary to produce a well-fitting crown. For fixed bridgework these steps are done on each and every anchor tooth, with the additional and sometimes difficult requirement that all prepared teeth be properly aligned (otherwise the final bridge will not go on). After the teeth are prepared and impressions taken, a temporary bridge is placed. At the next visit the dentist tries in the crowns and X-rays them to make sure they fit. Another impression is taken so that the crowns and the false teeth can be soldered together. Usually the dentist sees the patient at least twice more; once to try in the soldered bridge and once to cement the completed work. Many dentists like to temporarily cement the permanent bridge. We rarely do this because a well-fitting bridge can be almost impossible to remove even with temporary cement holding it in. But the soft temporary cement ultimately dissolves out and allows decay to get under the crowns. We believe that if the bridge fits properly it should be cemented permanently, and if it doesn't fit, having the patient wear it with temporary cement won't get it to fit (although it may get the patient used to wearing a poorly fitted restoration).

We have described the most popular method of producing a fixed bridge, but it is not the only way. Different techniques combine some visits and utilize shortcuts that can still produce good results, but too often they lead to defective bridgework. A dentist who is intent on saving time and who sees something wrong with his work may elect to ignore the imperfection and save himself the inconvenience of redoing some of his work. The result can only be a bridge that will not serve as well as it should. Too much is at stake to rush fixed bridgework. Quality dentists prefer methods such as we have outlined, in which each step is carefully checked before going on to the next step.

MARYLAND BRIDGES (RESIN-BONDED BRIDGES)

Bonding has revolutionized much of dentistry, and fixed bridgework is no exception. Using the bonding techniques we described in Chapter 9, dentists can actually bond metal to the teeth. A Maryland bridge (named after the University of Maryland where it was introduced) is also known as a resin-bonded bridge because bonding technology is used to anchor one or more missing teeth into the mouth. Instead of grinding down the anchor teeth for crowns, as is done in conventional fixed bridgework, the dentist takes only a small amount of enamel off the inside of the anchor teeth, requiring no anesthesia. An impression is taken and the lab produces a finished bridge, made of a steel alloy, that is bonded onto the roughed-up tooth structure. A resin-bonded bridge requires far less time and is far less expensive than a regular fixed bridge. Unfortunately, these types of bridges have not shown good results, many of them falling out in a few years. But for patients with serious medical problems or very young people missing permanent teeth, a Maryland bridge can be an excellent way of temporarily replacing teeth with a nonremovable bridge. It is also useful for splinting (tying together) periodontally weakened teeth.

Dr. Poorwork makes a lot of Maryland bridges. They are cheap enough to attract his patients and require little time and only a small lab fee. In the hands of a Poorwork this type of bridge is likely to lead to disastrous results. We've seen many patients with extensive decay and periodontal disease around Poorwork resin-bonded bridges.

Dr. Fraud often places resin-bonded bridges but charges the patient's union or insurance company for a conventional bridge. When such patients have come to us and we have applied for permission to construct a permanent fixed bridge, we've often been told by the insuring agency that the patient's former dentist had already received reimbursement for this work. Patients have told us time and again that they were told they had to sign the insurance form *before* their dentist would do the work, so they didn't know what had been put on their signed insurance forms. Being required to sign your forms before the work is done is one of the trademarks of Dr. Fraud.

We strongly recommend conventional fixed bridgework to replace missing permanent teeth. Make sure your dentist takes enough time and care to produce a successful bridge.

DENTAL IMPLANTS

One of the ways a missing tooth can be replaced is by placing an artificial "root" in the jawbone. This replacement root is called an implant. Implants have been around for a long time, but until recently the old-style implants were almost always rejected by the body with disastrous results. The problem was that there was insufficient animal research done by the early implant promoters, so it was the patients who were actually experimented on. And they paid a high fee for the dubious privilege, while the results were not accurately reported by the implant dentists. The dentists who did these implants claimed fabulous success, while the surgeons and general dentists who had to treat the consequences and complications of the failing implants reported horrible failures. One wag commented that implant research was performed on animals only after experimenting for years on humans, for a profit.

The answer was supplied by research done in Sweden by an orthopedic surgeon. Experimenting with various materials, he found that pins made of titanium seemed actually to attach themselves to bone. Years of research refined the technique, and the FDA approved these Swedish implants (commonly called Bränemark implants) for use in replacing missing teeth.

Today there are a host of Bränemark-like implants. They are cylindrical and made of or plated with titanium. The implant, placed in the jawbone, can accept a variety of differently shaped parts called abutments, which protrude through the gum. They can serve as an anchor for a new tooth, a "snap-on" kind of partial denture clip, a magnetic attachment, or a number of other innovative and useful devices. These new implants have an impressive success rate, but some failures are being noted as time goes on. Suffice it to say that implants, when properly planned and placed in the lower jaw, show excellent long-range success. Implants of the upper jaw are considerably less successful, but with careful case selection and execution they can be a valuable service.

Implant surgery is most often done in at least two stages. During the first surgery, the jawbone itself is exposed and holes are carefully drilled in the bone. The implants are then either lightly tapped, gently screwed, or simply placed in the hole. The gums are then sutured up, entirely covering the implants, and the patient is sent home to heal. The second surgery takes place after three to six months. The surgeon uncovers and exposes the implant, screws a metal piece called a healing cap into the implant, and again sends the patient home. If the implants are successfully "married" to the jawbone, a few weeks later the dentist places the type of restoration originally planned. This sounds complicated, and it is, but it's surprisingly painless. We've seen very few complications with this technique, and our patients have had minimal discomfort.

Implants have a number of advantages and a few disadvantages. Implants allow the permanent replacement of teeth without the conventional method of drilling and preparing the surrounding teeth for crowns. Or, if there are few or no natural teeth remaining, implants allow patients to hold full and partial dentures securely while still being able to remove the dentures for cleaning. And they are the only answer for people who have lost all their teeth and cannot wear a denture, or for people who have lost so many teeth that a conventional fixed bridge cannot be made.

On the other hand, they're time-consuming, often taking more than a year to complete. They're expensive, costing from $750 to $1,500 per implant, just for the surgery, without counting the cost of the replacement restoration, which can be considerable.

Not everyone can have implants. Many people, especially those who've been missing a lot of teeth for a very long time, don't have sufficient bone or the quality of bone necessary for implants. Some dentists want the patient to have a CT scan done to evaluate the amount and quality of the jawbone.

If you don't have enough quality bone, the surgeon may be able to build up the bone with bone taken from other areas or with techniques to move sensitive nerves or sinus cavities. These procedures are not without potential complications, such as permanent loss of feeling on part of the face or lips, but they can make possible an otherwise impossible case. Sometimes the negative side effects of the surgery outweighs the positive effects of the implants. This is especially true of surgery to move the nerves. A number of patients end up with chronic pain following this type of surgery. We strongly advise that you get a second opinion whenever extensive surgery is contemplated.

IMPLANT PROBLEMS

Implants are not trouble-free. They require meticulous upkeep and routine periodic checkups. And they can fail, even the new titanium implants. In most cases, the failing implant becomes loose but not infected and is easily removed. So you're no worse off than you were before you had the procedure, except for the expense. Often, you can have a new implant placed in a different location immediately, or you can wait a year or so, after the bone has healed, and have a new implant placed in the same location.

Many surgeons place more than the minimum number of implants required for a given case so that if one fails it can be removed, and the dental restoration constructed on the implants will still have enough support. This is something you should discuss with your dentist before any work is started.

A major problem with implants is that some dentists are unqualified to perform this service, particularly the surgery. There is no recognized specialty in implants, and some dentists have taken only a weekend seminar or even simply viewed a videotape before drilling into people's jaws. The surgery requires high levels of skill and experience. We recommend that you get as much information as you can beforehand. Write to the American Dental Association, 211 East Chicago Avenue, Chicago, IL 60611 and request information. Talk to patients who've had implants done in the office you're contemplating using. Find out exactly what kind and make of implant is going to be used, and don't be afraid to get a second opinion. Most important, make sure the dentist has the proper experience doing implants before you allow yourself to be operated on.

15. Orthodontics

*

O rthodontic treatment corrects or stabilizes the position of the teeth, usually through the use of adjustable braces. Most orthodontic patients are children, but the treatment of adults is also feasible, though more difficult. Some general practitioners do orthodontic work, but most of it is done by specialists who limit their practices to orthodontics.

Orthodontics is ridden with controversy. Cases for which one school prescribes a certain type of treatment are analyzed and treated in an entirely different fashion by another school. There are no convincing statistics to demonstrate the superiority of one method over another, and there may never be, because it is almost impossible to isolate and evaluate all the variables. This is the theoretical climate in which orthodontics is practiced, and there is no hope of soon resolving the controversies.

Cynics have said that the orthodontic need of children is in direct proportion to their parents' ability and willingness to pay, and, indeed, orthodontic treatment is much more common in affluent areas. It is true that very few people have a "perfect" bite, which allows considerable leeway for the unethical orthodontist to prescribe unneeded treatment, since a less-than-perfect bite does not necessarily mean that treatment is indicated. Many parents, terrified that they may not be doing everything they should for their children, actually do them a disservice when they arrange for unnecessary orthodontic work, and some orthodontists are too willing to accept patients who do not need their attention.

In orthodontics, aesthetics is the name of the game. Despite the claims of some orthodontists, there is no evidence that a "bad bite" leads to disease, pain, or improper function in the future. We have seen patients whose bites deviate massively from the "norm" and yet have no disease, discomfort, or trouble eating. In almost every case, the purpose of orthodontic treatment is to make the patient look better, period. Orthodontics will not prevent TMJ, or headaches, or gum disease, or improper nutrition. But it can make the patient look a great deal better, and this is always a major consideration. If the patient looks all right, has a decent smile and profile, there should be no need for orthodontics.

A competent and honest orthodontist can give the patient the best evaluation of whether treatment is desirable and what results can be expected. The best guide to the integrity of the orthodontist is the patient's conscientious dentist, who is in a position to evaluate the specialist's way of working and results. It can also help to talk with other patients of the orthodontist.

In the typical child the development of the dentition follows certain usual patterns that lead to a normal adult dentition with normal occlusion (bite). By normal we mean within acceptable limits of appearance. As the teeth come in and take their place in the developing dental arch, the growth and development of the jawbone keep pace with and are profoundly affected by the growth and positioning of the teeth. (Chapter 18 details this process.) If for any reason some teeth are prevented from taking their correct positions in the dental arch, the whole developmental mechanism of the jaws can be upset, often with unpleasant results for the formation of the face and profile. Preventive and corrective orthodontic treatment, by effecting better positioning of the teeth, often improves the development of the jaw and thus leads to greatly improved appearance. Teeth that are not crowded are also easier to clean and keep healthy.

The results of treatment can be dramatic. A child whose facial appearance is marred by a faulty dentition may show an astounding improvement in appearance as relatively simple orthodontic treatment progresses. Dramatic changes in profile and facial form often accompany the realignment of the teeth and jaws. Favorable results of this sort have the most positive effect on the child's developing personality; it is no exaggeration to say that effective orthodontic therapy can profoundly affect the child's entire life. Perhaps it is this realization that makes people willing to pay the high fees involved.

HOW ORTHODONTICS WORKS

It is the unique properties of the alveolar bone of the jaws that make it possible to reposition the teeth. The alveolar bone is the part of the jawbone that directly surrounds the roots of the teeth. Pressure in certain directions, applied through the teeth to the alveolar bone, results in resorption of the bone, which is an actual dissolution; the bone elements are decalcified and carried off by the bloodstream. Yet force applied to alveolar bone in *other* directions can serve to strengthen it.

These same properties of alveolar bone can cause problems in adult life; resorption of the bone in response to certain pressures, chemical as well as mechanical, leads to periodontal disease, the most common cause of tooth loss. In fact, a common feature of periodontal treatment is the reshaping of dentition to relieve destructive pressures on the bone while chewing. But the orthodontist is able to relocate teeth by exploiting these properties of alveolar bone. By the use of orthodontic appliances, usually braces, the doctor creates a controlled pressure that causes a controlled resorption of the alveolar bone. As the bone is resorbed in response to the pressures generated by the braces, the tooth, guided by the appliance, moves into the space created by the resorption. New bone then forms behind the tooth to fill in the space that has been vacated. This explains how the orthodontist can seem to move a tooth bodily through a block of solid bone.

These procedures are not without risk, and care must be taken by the doctor. In a young child, healing is quick and efficient, and new bone is rapidly formed to replace the resorbed bone. But as the individual gets older this process becomes less efficient, and the teeth must be moved more slowly, lest the new bone not form and the bony defect become permanent, seriously weakening the tooth. In adults particularly, tooth movement should be done slowly and deliberately. Another risk associated with rapid tooth movement is resorption of the root of the tooth, leaving less root to hold the tooth in place. A competent orthodontist takes great care not to use excessive force or obtain too-rapid tooth movement.

SPECIFIC TREATMENTS

A great variety of treatments are used. There are full-banded fixed appliances, generally considered best for a typical case; removable braces, which are cheaper and easier to use but considered less effective (although we have seen some successful cases done this way); "functional" appliances, which are removable devices intended to put pressure on the muscles of the mouth, with the muscles then affecting growth of the jaws; appliances that attach to the head, and others that extend outside the mouth. Some orthodontists recommend, for some cases, "serial" extractions of the baby teeth; some cases are treated with extractions of permanent teeth; some schools of treatment condemn *any* extractions. And so the controversies rage. Orthodontics can be a mystery, even to some orthodontists. But most orthodontic treatment is relatively successful, because competent orthodontists are sufficiently flexible to adapt treatment to the particular demands of the case.

SPECIAL CONCERNS FOR CHILDREN'S TEETH

Another reason for orthodontic treatment is the premature loss of baby teeth (see Chapter 18). A baby tooth lost too soon cannot serve to maintain enough space for the permanent tooth to conveniently grow in, and the permanent tooth might then come in crowded out of position. Some habits of childhood can cause malocclusion (poor positioning of teeth). These include thumb-sucking, chewing pencils or teddy bears, and certain habitual movements of cheek, lip, and tongue that can produce pressures causing teeth to shift. The use of pacifiers has been condemned by some authorities. But none of these is necessarily harmful. Some youngsters go through stages of thumb-sucking, or even pacifiers with no harm to the teeth, while the teeth of many other children react unfavorably. No measures need be taken if there is no sign of developing malocclusion, but if such evidence is present it is time to consult the dentist.

A program for prevention of malocclusion in a child calls for good care of the primary teeth so that none are lost prematurely, and the discovery, analysis, and correction of harmful habits. If a baby tooth is lost prematurely, a space-maintainer appliance can keep open the space needed for the permanent tooth. But sometimes even the most enlightened actions of parent and dentist cannot prevent malocclusion, and orthodontic treatment may be necessary.

If you are concerned about your child's bite, the first thing to do is discuss things with your family dentist, who often finds that there is really no problem after all. The new front teeth rarely come in straight, and we have had to reassure many a panicky parent that these teeth will straighten themselves out as the jaw develops. If the family dentist spots a problem, he can judge whether a consultation with an orthodontist is in order or whether the child can wait some more to see how things develop. If treatment is recommended, and you are concerned about fees, frank discussions with the orthodontist and the family dentist may help you decide whether the benefits will be worth their cost.

Orthodontics has its risks, and parents contemplating treatment for their child ought to be aware of them. First of all, there is no assurance that the treatment will be successful. Even apparently successful treatment sometimes relapses in a few years, the old malocclusion returning. To head off relapse, some children have to wear a retainer appliance at night. And there are Poorworks among orthodontists. Teeth moved too quickly, with too much force, can cause resorbed roots and damaged jawbone. Sometimes treatment brings little improvement. And sometimes the child is not cooperative and does not use the appliances as directed; in such cases failure can be expected. But all in all, the potential benefits of needed and proper orthodontic treatment far outweigh the possible drawbacks.

The careful orthodontist takes a number of precautions during the course of treatment. Bands made around the teeth to support and anchor braces should fit snugly, and they should be carefully cemented to prevent decay under the bands. New adhesive techniques can be used, which utilize the acid-etch bonding method with plastic brackets. (See Chapter 9.) Metal bands are not used in this method, with a more aesthetic result, but it is not suitable for every tooth or every case. In some neighborhoods "designer" braces, made of various colors, are the rage, silly though it seems. Even a well-made appliance is an efficient food collector and may become an indirect cause of decay. You therefore may need to supervise your child's brushing. At intervals in treatment the orthodontist may remove all appliances in order to permit the family dentist to check for decay.

Intelligent cooperation among parent, specialist, and dentist provides the best chance to realize the full potential benefits of orthodontic treatment.

ORTHODONTICS AND TMJ

It has been pretty well established by now that so-called TMJ pain has nothing to do with the bite, the way the teeth come together. But some orthodontists are claiming, without proof, that orthodontic treatment can prevent or cure TMJ problems. We feel that these claims amount to quackery.

Related to this are claims that have been made against orthodontists that their treatment has changed the bite and caused TMJ problems. Once again, there is no scientific support to these claims. (See Chapter 20.)

16. Cosmetic Dentistry

*

Every American dentist has been trained to make restorations that not only restore health and function but also look good. Some dentists call themselves "cosmetic dentists" and claim that they take special efforts to make their restorations aesthetic. But there is no recognized specialty in cosmetics. Every good dentist is capable of getting excellent aesthetic results. New restorative techniques make superior aesthetic results easier to achieve.

BONDING

Stained and discolored teeth can be covered with tooth-colored composite materials easily and without great expense; the result is generally called "bonding." Bondings provide a more economical solution to aesthetic problems that previously required more costly crowns and jackets.

Bonding has greatly influenced dentistry in the last twenty-five years. Strictly speaking, bonding is a chemical adhesive technique that allows us to attach materials to teeth in ways that were impossible with previous methods. Nowadays, dentists bond not only white composite front fillings but also silver fillings and gold crowns, inlays, and posts. Bonding allows the dentist to conserve more tooth structure, prevent sensitivity by sealing the teeth better, and produce better cosmetic results. Although there are distinct advantages to bonding, the technique is very sensitive and requires time and meticulous attention to detail. A small amount of saliva contamination can undermine a bonded restoration, but with good technique a very fine result can be achieved. (A more detailed description of bonding techniques can be found in Chapter 9.)

A few years ago there was a vast difference in the quality of a silver filling in a back tooth and a composite, tooth-colored filling. The silver filling was far stronger, resisted wear, produced a clearer

X-ray image so decay could be detected more easily, lasted far longer, and cost much less. The bonded composite filling materials have been improved to the point that they now are almost as good as silver fillings. But they are much more difficult to do, take much more time, do not last as long, and are much more expensive. Silver fillings for back teeth are still preferred, but the composite materials are catching up.

BLEACHING

Dentists have been bleaching teeth in their offices for years, with variable results. Bleaching is an involved process and should be supervised by the dentist to ensure that the patient is not injured by the caustic bleaching agent. The public has recently been exposed to a flurry of advertising for at-home tooth-bleaching agents. The safety and effectiveness of the nonsupervised use of these products are questionable at best. At-home products have a much lower concentration of bleach, but nonetheless they may be dangerous if too strong, or not effective if too weak.

At-home bleaching products received through a dentist's office and supervised by a dentist are more likely to be the proper strength. The dentist takes impressions and provides a custom-made plastic tray to hold a safe amount of bleach against specific surfaces of the teeth. (This way you are not likely to swallow bleach.) It usually takes about three weeks of at-home treatment to achieve the desired results.

But none of these techniques are backed by proper studies to show that they are safe and effective in the long term. The most common bleaching agent is concentrated hydrogen peroxide. It is called an oxygenating agent because it works by releasing oxygen, which reacts with the enamel to make it a lighter color. The American Dental Association cites early studies that link long-term use of oxygenating agents with cancer. They are also linked to side effects such as tooth sensitivity, gum irritation, and stomach upset. While close supervision by a dentist reduces the chances of being injured by the caustic bleaching agent, even dentist-supervised tooth bleaching occasionally produces erratic results. It is interesting that these materials and techniques, even those intended to be used under close dental supervision, are promoted as *cosmetics,* not as drugs or medical treatments; this is to avoid scrutiny by the Food and Drug Administration. Considering the present status of bleaching procedures, we recommend caution, at least until evidence of long-term safety and effectiveness appears in the scientific literature.

CERAMICS

Recent progress in technology has brought ceramic crowns and inlays back to some level of popularity, mostly in "cosmetic" dental practices. In the past these restorations did not live up to expectations, leaking, decaying at the margins, and breaking far too often. While they have been quite successful in certain situations (for example, all-porcelain jackets on front teeth), research indicates that ceramic materials are brittle, not strong enough, and subject to stress failure over time.

COMPOSITE INLAYS

The lab-processed composite inlay is a rather new and useful technique that is gaining widespread popularity. Composite materials when lab-processed are very durable, color stable, wear resistant, easy to handle, and extremely beautiful. They can be readily bonded to the tooth and are useful where too much tooth is missing to do a good silver or composite filling but where a crown would remove even more tooth structure. The excellent bonding potential of composite allows a conservative tooth preparation and seemingly gives a reasonably good prognosis. Time will tell how successful this attractive technique will be.

17. Oral Hygiene: Products and Gimmicks

*

To begin this chapter, we offer you the candid testimony of the Duchess in Gilbert and Sullivan's *The Gondoliers*:

> *I write letters blatant*
> *On medicines patent*
> *And use any other you mustn't—*

> *And vow my complexion*
> *Derives its perfection*
> *From somebody's soap—which it doesn't—*

Knowledge of dental disease and its prevention and treatment has become so comprehensive that with today's information, intelligently applied, virtually no one should suffer significant loss of teeth. Even when disease is advanced, in most cases remarkable results can be obtained, *provided there is full patient cooperation*. This is crucial; the dentist is nearly helpless when confronting the single most important cause of dental disease—poor oral hygiene. Even dentistry by Dr. Goodwork may not succeed in a mouth that is neglected and shows unrepentant poor oral hygiene. Today's dentist, fully aware of this problem, should be willing to spend as much time as is necessary to teach patients the principles and methods of proper home care. And he should be paid for this most important service.

Although losing one's teeth is not as serious as losing a hand or a foot, people who lose their teeth are indeed handicapped. Dentures are only fair substitutes for natural teeth, and research indicates that older people with their own teeth eat better and feel better, and actually seem and act younger than do their contemporaries who have lost their teeth. Today good dental health is within the reach of everyone. Even for people with "bad teeth," people whose teeth are uncommonly susceptible to decay (whether because of genetics, oral chemistry, or the constitution of the teeth), conscientious oral hygiene and timely, excellent dentistry will almost always triumph, with the result that such individuals need not lose teeth. And in the case of the decay-free but periodontal-disease-prone person with "good teeth but bad gums," routine periodontal care by the dentist—not a Poorwork—will prevent a sad fate.

The TV commercial shows a lovely young woman talking about her daddy, a dentist, who had never before given her advice about her teeth (not much of a close-knit family this). But now, finally, the chain of silence has been broken, and Daddy has advised her to use a certain baking soda and peroxide dentifrice. And off she purrs, radiating a dazzling smile.

The importance of oral hygiene has been a major theme of Madison Avenue. Relying on its most hallowed principle, that a little knowledge is a profitable thing, the advertising industry has enriched itself and some of its clients by building up and exploiting the public's fears of poor oral hygiene (offending breath, unsightly smile) and the advantages (social acceptance and romance) of a clean, "sweet-smelling" mouth. Yet after years of watching and reading commercials for dental products, only one advertisement stands out as telling the complete truth about an oral hygiene topic: An ad from a major toothpaste manufacturer clearly stated that there is no evidence that baking soda and peroxide do any good for the mouth. Every other ad we have seen has, either directly or by implication, sought to mislead the public. And, sad to say, that one refreshingly honest ad did not run very long.

Here, to clear the air before we go any farther, is the truth about teeth and dental products:

The natural color of adult teeth is not white, and it is harmful to attempt to scrub teeth until they get white. Harsh scouring to whiten teeth, with one of the so-called whitening abrasive toothpastes (often marketed to smokers), not only can cause severe damage but actually causes the teeth to become darker in color. The outer shell of a tooth, called the enamel, is lighter in color than the inner layer, the dentin. As the enamel is worn thin by overenthusiastic brushing with abrasive toothpaste, the darker-colored dentin shows through, darkening the tooth.

Teeth should be brushed gently, with mildly abrasive tooth-paste.

The natural color of a tooth is yellowish, ranging from a gray-yellow to a light reddish-yellow. This color range holds for all races. Some toothpastes contain a solution of hydrogen peroxide and are marketed as whitening or bleaching toothpastes. Experts warn that self-bleaching may not be effective and might be dangerous. In order to lower the danger (and the possibility of litigation), the manufacturers have decreased the concentration of hydrogen peroxide bleach to a level that is unlikely to be effective for anything but advertising hype.

It is the toothbrush, not the toothpaste, that does the important work. Therefore, the choice of toothpaste makes little difference, so long as it is not harmful, for instance, because of being too abrasive. Gentle toothpaste is helpful in that the detergents, mild scouring abrasives, and foaming agents help carry off the debris dislodged by the brush. Baking soda and peroxide are oxygenating agents that can upset the ecological balance of saliva (see below). As the ad said, there is no evidence that they do any good.

The list of ingredients on toothpaste packages is instructive. The only "active ingredient" listed is fluoride, which is the only ingredient that has been proved to do some good.

No mouthwash, toothpaste, or lozenge can cure mouth odors. Indeed, commercial mouthwashes that contain a large volume of alcohol may be dangerous if used excessively (one popular mouthwash has more alcohol than wine). It is true that most cases of what advertisers call bad breath are caused by conditions in the mouth, but the most a mouthwash or other product can do is briefly mask the odor. Meanwhile the condition that causes the odor freely attacks the gums behind the masking counterodor of the "antihalitosis" product. Any commercial over-the-counter mouthwash, if used consistently, may destroy the ecological balance of the bacteria and chemicals in the mouth. New, unforeseen difficulties may result, and the old difficulty, for which the mouthwash was mistakenly used, is likely to become worse than ever.

There are no such things as "detergent foods." Crunchy foods such as apples are often described as being able to clean the teeth by removing plaque. Some government publications have even made this claim. But although coarse foods may exercise the teeth and gums, they are not a substitute for proper oral hygiene. Studies on a variety of foods have shown that under the very best circumstances chewing may help clean the upper third of the teeth. But the critical areas where diseases of the gums and decay proliferate, under the gums, are unaffected by so-called detergent foods.

Plaque is the major cause of dental disease. The purpose of oral hygiene is to remove as much plaque and debris from the mouth as possible. It is essential to interfere with plaque formation before it produces sufficient acids and bacterial by-products to destroy the teeth and gums. (See Chapters 9 and 10.) Oral debris has only one source, food. Small particles of food that collect between the teeth, along the gums, and elsewhere in the mouth are digested by the ever-present bacteria and start to ferment. The saliva is able to control only some of these bacterial by-products. It is under these conditions that dental plaque and tartar (which is calcified plaque) are formed, and this leads to tooth decay and gum disease. Removing the food residues, which the bacteria digest, from the mouth promptly after eating reduces the amount of bacterial acids and toxins to a minimum, but this is easier said than done. Even though there is a direct correlation between oral hygiene efforts and a reduction in oral disease, the methods of oral hygiene, even when applied conscientiously, are not always completely effective.

The mouth has a tendency to keep itself clean, but food residues collect in the most difficult areas for the tongue and saliva to reach: between the teeth, in the deep grooves of the back teeth, and along the gumline. Even the toothbrush often has difficulty reaching these most important areas. Special attention must therefore be paid to these areas during cleaning. The amount and thickness of the saliva, position of the teeth, size of the mouth, and action of the tongue and cheeks all contribute to the ease or difficulty of keeping a particular mouth clean. Consequently, some rare people can have excellent oral hygiene with very little effort, but most of us have to take the time to learn proper methods of home care and take adequate time, each day, to maintain our oral health.

Brush your gums. Food and plaque collect in the gum-edge

area. Many cavities start here, especially in older people whose salivary flow has decreased, and this is where tartar begins to form. Over the years various methods of brushing have been proposed. The once-popular hard-bristle toothbrush is no longer recommended. It is much better to use a soft-bristle nylon brush that is less abrasive and vibrate the bristles right into the gum-tooth junction. We believe that as long as you brush without excessive pressure and don't abrade, puncture, or otherwise irritate the oral tissues, one technique of brushing is probably as good as another, but try to cover every surface of every tooth, especially at the gum line. Electric toothbrushes, carefully used, do an excellent job. Some of the newer electric toothbrushes use high-frequency "ultrasonic" vibrations to remove debris. They seem quite effective and cannot do any damage. But good results can be obtained using a plain old manual toothbrush. It takes some degree of dexterity to accomplish this. An advantage of the electric toothbrush is that less skill and hence less practice are needed to achieve the desired result. The best way to learn proper toothbrushing methods is to ask your dentist or hygienist to demonstrate them.

Various toothbrush manufacturers are making claims about the superiority of the shape of their brushes. But the oddly-shaped brushes are no better, and probably less effective than the old, simple, classic straight toothbrush. Incidentally, a toothbrush should be discarded once the bristles seem deformed, usually three or four times a year.

The oral hygiene of young children presents special problems. The major difficulty is that they lack the dexterity and commitment to brush their teeth effectively. Furthermore, the eating habits of the typical child are likely to leave food residues in the mouth much of the time. Milk, formula, or juice given to bottle-fed infants may help produce decay. It is not wise to permit a baby to fall asleep with a bottle in his mouth, or to allow a baby to suck on a bottle all day long. Children should try to brush their own teeth but should be assisted in brushing by their parents until about the age of six. (See Chapter 18.)

Brush after meals. Most people brush at the wrong times. The bacteria that live in the mouth need time to produce sufficient acid and toxins to damage the mouth. Therefore, brushing should be timed to interrupt this cycle. In most people this requires a thorough and meticulous cleaning twice a day. Many people who believe they exercise careful oral hygiene make the serious mistake of brushing as soon as they wake up before breakfast. Their mouths are clean for only the few minutes between the morning brushing and breakfast; the rest of the day food residues are doing their nasty work in the mouth. An effective brushing schedule is to brush carefully *after* breakfast and before retiring at night. This way the mouth is clean of food residue most of the time.

THE TRUTH ABOUT TOOTHPASTE

The extravagant promotion of chemical additives has always been popular with toothpaste manufacturers. Over the last thirty years these have included carbamide (urea), chlorophyll, hexachorophene, chloroform, baking soda, peroxide, sanguinaria, "anti-tartar" formulas, and various forms of fluoride. A lot of "research" has attempted to back up some of these claims. The results of such research, it may not be surprising to learn, have been much more favorable to the product when the research was paid for by the manufacturer than when it was done independently. Recently an FDA advisory panel found no convincing evidence that baking soda or sanguinaria is effective against plaque accumulation or gum disease.

Some toothpaste manufacturers make the popular claim that their product has an "anti-tartar" formula, implying that it can remove calculus or slow the growth of new calculus. *Any toothpaste,* used in conjunction with a toothbrush, accomplishes this. While some studies show that certain chemical toothpaste additives do indeed help in removing tartar that is *above* the gum line, they don't help with disease-causing under-the-gum tartar. Gum inflammation, a major sign of periodontal disease, is not reduced by the use of these "anti-tartar" toothpastes. Furthermore, some of these chemical additives *interfere with enzymatic activity of the saliva,* and questions have been raised about the long-term safety of using these formulations. Since their contribution to oral health is trivial at best, and since there are doubts about their safety, we do not recommend their use.

Of course fluoride, usually the only active ingredient listed on the toothpaste container, does help reduce decay, but it is much more effective when taken internally, from a fluoridated water supply, than when applied topically. We recommend you always use a fluoridated toothpaste; like chicken soup, it cannot do any harm and may do some good (see the section on fluoridation for more information).

The other ingredients in a toothpaste are, commonly: an abrasive, binding agents to hold the paste together, sudsing agents, moisturizers, flavoring agents, coloring, and water. Some toothpastes claim that they're "natural." This implies that they are safer than other toothpastes, but this is nonsense, pandering to those poorly informed people who think something must be good if it is "natural." Of course, whether or not it is natural is not the point: What is important is whether or not it is safe and effective. All toothpastes that have been accepted by the American Dental Association are safe, in the sense that they are not too abrasive. Extra money spent on a "natural" dentifrice is thrown away. Some toothpastes are specifically targeted for people with sensitive teeth, but we have found their results to be inconsistent.

OTHER METHODS OF ORAL HYGIENE

There are many aids to cleaning the mouth besides toothbrush and toothpaste. The most important is a glass of water. Thorough, forceful rinsing of the mouth after brushing is a must. Cavity-prone individuals can also be helped considerably by strong rinsing with water after snacks or drinks; of course brushing, if possible, is even better. Ordinary water is also the best mouthwash and should be the only mouthwash you ever use, unless you have a diagnosed condition that requires specific medication.

Dental floss, dental tape, and toothpicks are the best-known mechanical complements to brushing. Dental floss is a strong thread that is passed between the teeth to loosen and remove debris wedged between them. Dental tape is a thicker form of floss. A toothpick, if properly used, can be handy for removing plaque from around the teeth. The Perio-Aid is a useful device that holds the pointed ends of a round toothpick so that you can more easily manipulate the toothpick into difficult-to-get-to places. Stim-U-

Dents are over-the-counter toothpicks with a sophisticated design. Some dentists and periodontists recommend them routinely for therapeutic home care. There are also a number of special small conical brushes, as well as floss threaders for getting floss under the soldered joints of fixed bridges. Most people should floss once a day.

Water-irrigating devices such as the Water-Pik represent a significant advance in home oral hygiene technology. The strong pulsating stream of water loosens debris, dilutes acids and toxins, stimulates the gums, and oxygenates the areas under the gum line where bacteria breed, thereby slowing their growth. To use these devices properly, place the nozzle tip firmly touching the teeth and the gum at the gum line between the two teeth, and spray the stream of water *straight through,* not into the gum and not toward the lip. The force of the spray can be kept low to moderate. If misused, these devices can hasten the dissolution of the cement seal of poorly made crowns and inlays; this effect does not occur with well-made restorations having sound margins. All in all, it is best to use an oral irrigating device under the guidance of a good dentist or experienced dental hygienist. Water-irrigating devices take much less time to use than floss, and some authorities feel that using them is superior to flossing. But most authorities still prefer flossing.

The usefulness of toothpastes and mouthwashes can be understood only in relation to the natural chemistry of the mouth. The chief factor is the saliva (which is more fully discussed in Chapter 6). The importance of saliva in maintaining good oral hygiene cannot be overestimated. Though the mouth is host to more than eighty known varieties of microorganisms, they tend, always under the influence of the saliva, to keep one another in balance and under control so that they do not lead to harmful infections even after oral traumas such as pizza burns or cheek biting or even tooth extractions.

Suppose that we flooded this unique environment with a strong chemical that kills off a good many of the microorganisms normally found in the mouth. The surviving types of microorganisms would then be able to proliferate. And this is exactly what happens when certain mouthwashes are used frequently. Just for example, continual use of any peroxide mouthwash to "treat" bleeding gums can lead to the proliferation of certain varieties of an ugly fungus that causes an infection picturesquely called black hairy tongue. If caught early, black hairy tongue clears up promptly once the peroxide mouthwash is discontinued (black hairy tongue can also be caused by overuse of systemic antibiotics).

Since germs were first implicated in the decay process and gum disease, it's been hoped that a medicine would be found that could inactivate those germs and prevent most dental disease. Research into vaccines, systemic drugs, and locally applied medications are ongoing. Within the last ten years a number of mouthwashes have been marketed with "antibacterial" claims. The only mouthwash with true efficacy requires a prescription and contains the FDA approved drug, chlorhexidine. In other countries chlorhexidine is available without a prescription, and there is pressure for the FDA to allow over-the-counter sales. Chlorhexidine mouthwashes are useful for plaque control, control of oral fungal infections, treatment of acute gum infection and seem to be helpful in treating canker sores. Its side effects are minor, the most noted being temporary staining of the teeth and tongue. This staining requires more frequent dental cleanings.

The use of any medicated mouthwash should be reserved for specific, rare conditions and should not be used for a prolonged period of time. Furthermore, mouthwashes should not be used except as directed by a dentist. Yet millions of Americans, prodded by persistent advertising, do use mouthwashes habitually, in some cases becoming reliant on them. Thus a new artificial chemical and microbiological balance is established which, unlike nature's balance, is extremely precarious and may easily be upset.

We are often asked about that "horrible morning taste" in the mouth. The healthy mouth quickly accommodates to the taste of a water rinse before breakfast and a brushing afterward, and stays much healthier. Mouths with genuinely foul tastes, which water does not dispel, probably suffer from gum disease and should receive appropriate treatment. (More information on this in the halitosis section, below.)

The over-the-counter mouthwashes and hydrogen peroxide rinses are not of value for anything but superficial plaque removal. We believe that, since they are not effective and may be harmful, you are best off rinsing with plain water. Mouthwashes touted as "prebrushing rinses" have not been shown to have benefits at all.

HALITOSIS

"Halitosis" is one of those words invented by an advertising copywriter that has since worked its way into common language. Halitosis, or bad breath, is a common problem on which Americans spend millions of dollars. Some dentists have even opened practices dedicated solely to curing bad breath. Most of us have tried over-the-counter mouthwashes that claim to prevent or minimize mouth odors. In 1994, *Consumer Reports* published the results of a test of fifteen mouthwashes. They found that for people who had their breath tested before and after eating garlic pizza, all the tested products worked for about ten minutes, and some were slightly effective after an hour, but "no product proved to be consistently better than any other. And at the end of two hours, they all had fairly little residual effect."

In healthy mouths, bad breath is caused by plaque accumulations; proper brushing and flossing corrects the problem. People with gum disease often suffer from halitosis. Smokers have a particular odor associated with cigarettes or cigars, and are also more prone to gum problems. A dry mouth, which could result from many causes including medications, age (older people produce less saliva), anemia, diabetes, emotional stress, mechanical blockage of the salivary ducts, damage due to irradiation, AIDS, multiple sclerosis, and diseases of the salivary glands, can also cause bad odors. And mouth breathing caused by allergies can lead to a dry and odorous mouth. Finally, eating certain foods such as garlic and onions causes a distinctive odor until the offending food is metabolized.

Attempting to mask the odors with mouthwashes or "breath mint" candies is a waste of time. Mouthwashes don't work, and "breath mints" are merely decay-producing candies. Proper treatment of mouth odors is aimed at eliminating their causes. Scrupulous oral hygiene, including brushing the back of the tongue, is the first step, since oral bacteria are the most frequent causative agents. Tobacco products should be discontinued, and not only for cosmetic reasons. A balanced, healthful diet is always a good idea. If a diagnosis of oral disease cannot be arrived at, and the dentist does detect the odor, then you should be referred to a physician for evaluation because unpleasant mouth odors can indicate diseases of the stomach or lungs. Some dentists are selling products that contain the compound chlorine dioxide with the claim that this cures halitosis. Chlorine dioxide is used as an algacide in swimming pools; there are no data to support its use orally as being safe and effective.

To summarize, a complete exam should be done, an accurate diagnosis made, and an appropriate treatment plan adopted for halitosis. This treatment plan will almost always involve cleaning up the mouth with scalings and cleanings, advanced periodontal treatment if needed, and, always, careful oral hygiene. If systemic disease is suspected, a medical referral should be given.

Mouthwashes and toothpastes cannot cure any type of halitosis, despite the solemn affirmations of the advertisers. All the products can do is mask the taste, odor, and discomfort for a brief period of time. It's like putting perfume on garbage; this can be particularly poignant when the garbage is in one's own mouth. The astringent and anesthetic action of the chemical agents in these preparations can give a diseased, foul-smelling mouth a temporary feeling of well-being, which is dangerous if you are thereby dissuaded from seeking proper treatment. Untreated, a destructive periodontal condition continues until crippling damage to the mouth results. Yet the advertisements still give the clear impression that the right way to treat problem gums, halitosis, and mouth discomfort is to use whatever toothpaste or mouthwash is being promoted. The patient who relies on the advertising industry for oral hygiene information is likely to pay dearly for this misplaced faith.

CONSUMER BEWARE

In 1991 the FDA ordered twenty manufacturers of bleaching products containing hydrogen or carbamide peroxide to stop marketing them until they were demonstrated to be safe and effective. A case had been reported of a boy who had permanently damaged his teeth by applying an over-the-counter bleaching product seven times a day. This gradually stripped the enamel from his teeth, causing them to darken. Unfortunately, toothpastes are not considered drugs but cosmetics and are therefore almost totally free from FDA oversight.

Dr. Poorwork also likes to have his patients use strong over-the-counter mouthwashes and special toothpaste formulations. This helps mask the neglect and the dreadful mouth tastes and odors rampant among Dr. Poorwork's patients. Dr. Quack gets into the act by selling "special," "natural," or "herbal" toothpastes and mouthwashes, finding another way to profit from his patients' lack of accurate information.

You may wonder how companies and advertising agencies can get away with fraudulent advertising. Aren't there laws to protect the consumer against misrepresentation and fraud? Such laws do exist, but the advertising copywriters circumvent these laws by never saying anything explicit about their products; they are content to misrepresent by suggestion and lack of full information. The ad never actually states that ABC Mouthwash cures halitosis; instead it says, "ABC keeps breath fresh for hours." Of course, the word "fresh" has no precise meaning. The lie is reinforced and greatly magnified by the TV ad showing the model's romantic success. The model brushes her teeth with the product and then is seen walking arm in arm with a handsome young man. Under our present laws such a vague but emotionally appealing suggestion cannot be legally challenged.

Occasionally the copywriters do overstep the boundaries of the law by making direct claims that are patently false. The government may then prosecute, but litigation can take years, and even after a manufacturer loses a case, it turns out that the penalties prescribed by law are no more than a slap on the wrist, measured against an advertising budget in the millions and millions more of profits generated by the fraudulent ads. The company is ordered not to repeat the offending advertisements so it comes up with a new campaign, complete with new lies. Meanwhile the understaffed and underfunded government agency struggles to prepare a new case against some other fraudulent advertiser. Such prosecutions get very little media attention. There is much to be said about advertising, but this should be enough to convince the reader that advertising copy and commercials are not reliable sources of information on oral hygiene—if they are a reliable source of information about anything at all.

We offer the wisdom of Confucius, who must have had a premonition of Madison Avenue in mind when he said: "The superior man knows what is right; the inferior man knows what will sell."

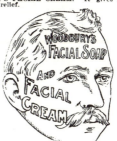
This 1897 dental journal ad typifies the lack of consumer protection before the FDA and FTC were established. Here a product is promoted as an effective cleaner, wrinkle remover, treatment for eczema, and toothpaste! (Illustration from *Items of Interest,* A Monthly Magazine of Dental Art, Science and Literature, September 1897.)

18. Children's Teeth

*

M any people still believe that children's teeth need not be cared for because they will be lost anyway. Or if they do receive treatment, the dentist need not spend much time with these "unimportant" teeth. These notions are not true, and the child victimized by these assertions may suffer for a lifetime because of them.

Children's teeth *are* important—vitally so. Not only do they help the child eat and speak, but even more important, they help the jaws to develop a normal and natural appearance and shape. The first teeth are called deciduous, primary, or baby teeth. They eventually are entirely replaced with what are called the secondary, or permanent teeth. The embryonic "buds" that form the teeth are present from the seventh week of pregnancy. The enamel of the tooth develops first; the root doesn't become complete until after the tooth has come in. That's why new teeth are a little bit loose.

The primary teeth start coming in when the child is around the age of six months (see chart, p. 154), and they must be properly cared for; they are essential for the development of the jaws and the permanent teeth. The premature loss of primary teeth usually leads to crowded and crooked permanent teeth. Therefore it's imperative that you start cleaning your children's teeth as soon as they erupt: a soft-bristled brush and warm water can be used with a six-month-old child.

By the age of three, children should be capable of brushing their own teeth. You should supervise them and brush any areas that weren't properly cleaned. A small dab of toothpaste can be used with toddlers, and flossing can also be utilized for children with tightly spaced primary teeth. Twice-a-day brushing habits, after breakfast and before bedtime, should be established early.

Continue to help your children with brushing up to the age of six or seven, making oral hygiene a daily and enjoyable routine. Children love attention and contact with their parents. Ordinary toothbrushes are fine, and electric toothbrushes are excellent and easy for children to use.

The most serious dental problem for young children is *baby bottle syndrome*. This occurs when a child is given a bottle filled with milk, formula, or fruit juice at bedtime, naptime, or for long periods during the day. The extended exposure of teeth to the sugars and acids in these drinks can cause extensive decay. Such decay can occur even with breast milk, since it also contains sugar. To prevent this syndrome, don't give your child a bottle at bedtime or naptime with anything other than water, and only if you have to, and always clean your child's teeth after each feeding.

A CHILD'S VISITS TO THE DENTIST

The American Academy of Pediatric Dentistry recommends that children be examined at the age of one. Most general dentists like to see a child before all the primary teeth have erupted, around the age of two and a half. It is difficult to work on a child who hasn't developed communication skills, so dentists prefer to work on children when they are a little older rather than younger.

Before you take your child to a dentist, we recommend that you first take him with you when you have a checkup so he can get used to the surroundings, sounds, smells, and people in a dental office. Avoid saying things such as, "If you're not good the dentist is going to give you a shot" or "It won't hurt." Your child probably never thought that it could hurt, so why put ideas in his head? Answer your child's questions honestly but without much detail. Let the dentist explain everything to the child. Confusion and fear are widespread causes of dental neglect, but careful handling by a dentist willing to spend the necessary time can settle the young child before the fears become entrenched. If your dentist doesn't treat children, you should find a pedodontist (a specialist in children's dental care).

Pedodontists usually design their offices to fulfill the psychological needs of children. Waiting rooms are filled with children's books and games. We've seen offices with jungle motifs so that the dental light looks like a giraffe; some even have computers and video games. A capable pedodontist uses special techniques to relieve a child's anxieties, and a terrified child can be turned into a cooperative patient who is never again afraid of going to a dentist. The pedodontist's goal is just that, and his fees, which may seem high, are justified by this achievement alone.

The psychological and other techniques employed by the pedodontist are exactly the same ones used by any dentist who treats children properly. When children come to a dentist for the first time, they are often filled with worries, usually because their knowledge of dentistry has been received from their friends. Their minds are filled with ideas of long needles and rattling drills. Parents, especially if they've had the misfortune to be patients of a Dr. Poorwork, have reinforced these fears with their own anxieties, either deliberately or inadvertently. Children are alert and perceptive, and they pick up attitudes from their parents without the parents ever suspecting. If the child has had a previous experience with Dr. Poorwork's speed-up dentistry, then the job of any future dentist will be that much harder because Dr. Poorwork has confirmed and cemented all the child's fears.

Children also have superb memories, and they cannot be fooled. They expect candid and honest behavior from the dentist. Because a good dentist knows children, he never attempts to deceive them. Dr. Poorwork hides an injection syringe or a drill or a forceps behind his back, sneaks up on the child patient, and WHAM! Poorwork will never be able to do proper work for the child; the child does not trust him enough to let him. What is worse, the child who has experienced such deception will be reluctant to accept dental care, making serious problems for future dentists.

Although children demand unrelenting honesty and candor from the dentist, they also offer an uncommon challenge and unusual rewards. Dentists can confidently expect to treat even the difficult child successfully, because, with modern techniques, including local anesthesia, the dental work will not hurt. And even though dentistry can be inconvenient, and it can be uncomfortable to hold your mouth open wide for a fairly long time period, there is no pain once the work is underway. That is the catch. The difficult child expects it to hurt, and the dentist must get the child to allow treatment so that he can understand that it doesn't hurt. Then the battle will be won.

But first the dentist must convince the child to allow some treatment, no matter how minor, to be accomplished. To make the task easier all around, the dentist begins with a simple goal, such as counting the teeth. After announcing the plan very clearly, the dentist must then actually count the child's teeth. If the child carries on and the dentist gives up, the lesson learned by the child is that he is in charge of the visit and can stop it any time by being uncooperative. So the dentist must persist; the child's future dental health depends on it. The dentist also needs the active help of the parent. Don't talk when the dentist is talking; not only will that confuse the child, but you will invariably say the wrong thing. Too often, after painstakingly preparing the child for a procedure, the parent blows everything by saying something like, "Don't worry, it won't hurt." Do what the dentist tells you to do. If the dentist says, "Mommy is going to leave now because you won't open your mouth," leave the room. The message to the child is that the dentist is someone even Mommy listens to. We've hardly ever failed to get an uncooperative child to behave if the parents help us.

With the average child, not particularly fearful, the approach will be the same but progress will be much faster. If the counting at the first visit goes smoothly, X rays may be taken and the child may be introduced to some of the tools a dentist uses. A face mirror given to the child to see what's happening is an absolute necessity. Children rarely fear what they can see. Of course, the dentist should never do anything without first fully explaining it to the child. In nearly every case in our recollection, even with difficult children, X rays and cleaning were accomplished by the end of the second visit, while fillings were usually started by the third visit, if not by the second.

TREATING CHILDREN'S TEETH

The treatment of children's teeth is essentially the same as for adult teeth, but there are some differences. Primary teeth have a different anatomy, besides being much smaller, with larger pulps and thinner enamel than permanent teeth. There is therefore less room and a smaller margin of error for the dentist drilling in primary teeth. The other important consideration is that the primary teeth will all fall out by around twelve years of age. It doesn't make sense to construct a major restoration for a tooth that will come out naturally in a short time, nor is it cost effective to fill a primary tooth that will soon be lost. The rule of thumb is not to fill a cavity if the tooth will be lost before the cavity starts to hurt. This saves time and money. The dentist is able to judge, from the X rays and the clinical appearance of the tooth, if the tooth should be treated or left alone until it falls out by itself.

Aside from these considerations, the treatment of baby teeth and permanent teeth is about the same. We believe that it is actually more difficult to fill a primary tooth than a similar cavity in a permanent tooth. A general dentist's fees for children's dentistry, therefore, should be comparable to the fees for adult dentistry.

Time, as we have stressed elsewhere in this book, is the indispensable key to success in all phases of dentistry, and children's dentistry is no exception.

In areas which do not have fluoride in the drinking water the use of fluoride supplements for very young children is essential. If your child is prone to cavities, stricter attention to diet and home care (less sugar and more brushing) is in order, and the use of an over-the-counter fluoride rinse could be helpful.

Parents often are concerned because of thumb-sucking or the use of a pacifier. Sucking is a normal instinct. Many infants start sucking their thumbs or using a pacifier within three months of birth. Thumb-sucking and pacifiers can cause the permanent teeth to grow in out of position if the child continues these habits past the age of five or six. Fortunately, most children discontinue these habits well before this age. If your child hasn't stopped, we recommend a program of positive reinforcement, with gold stars being given for every day that the child doesn't suck his thumb and a big prize being given if forty or fifty stars are earned. Sometimes peer pressure can help. (Do you want to be the only kid in class with your thumb in your mouth?) Appliances that have sharp spokes that stick into the thumb and torture kids aren't effective, nor is yelling at and punishing them. If worse comes to worst, the teeth are easier to fix than your child's psyche.

It's not surprising that in a country as affluent as the United States, the care and maintenance of children's teeth have a high priority. In many families, parents neglect their own needs in order to ensure that their children have a healthy and pain-free mouth. Even with all the widespread interest in children, we see a deplorable lack of knowledge and scandalous lack of quality care in the treatment of children's oral problems.

As an example, every year or so we hear the news that a child died in a dentist's office while undergoing routine dentistry, such as a few fillings, under general anesthesia. Children have this kind of dangerous anesthesia due to the parents' fears of dental pain and the dentist's assurances of safety. Often the child had been uncooperative in another dentist's chair, and the parents, being embarrassed, found a dentist, usually through an ad that says the dentist "caters to cowards," who will put their child "to sleep." They do this rather than finding a dentist who would take the time to relax the child's fears and convert the child to a cooperative patient. We believe that general anesthesia for filling teeth is absolutely unnecessary and should not be done, except in the case of a child with a medical problem that makes it impossible to do dentistry any other way, such as a child with seizures.

PRIMARY TEETH

When a child is born, the tooth "buds" for both the baby teeth and the permanent teeth are already present in the jaws. That's why it's so important to give a child fluoridated water, making the fluoride available for the formation of the teeth. Primary teeth are much smaller and whiter than the secondary teeth. Parents are often shocked when the permanent front teeth erupt and they compare them to the small bluish-white baby teeth. Although the new teeth are perfectly normal, they may appear huge and grotesque to the mother who's grown accustomed to seeing her child with only tiny, very white baby incisors. (For information about teething problems see Chapter 7.)

The primary teeth also guide the development of the jaws and maintain sufficient space for the permanent teeth. A baby tooth that is prematurely lost can no longer maintain the space required for the permanent tooth developing within the jaw, and when time comes for the permanent tooth to erupt there may not be enough room for it to come into place. That tooth may come in out of position, or it may stay in the jaw as an impacted tooth. If the permanent tooth forces its way into the mouth, it may cause overcrowding and a possible distortion of the entire dental arch. This is one of the most common causes of later orthodontic treatment, or braces, and is usually avoidable by taking care of the baby teeth.

From the standpoint of the ultimate development of the final form of the teeth and the jaws, the first permanent molars are by far the most important teeth in the mouth. They are keystones of the dental arch and their presence helps to correctly align the developing back teeth. But we have seen many children ten or eleven years old already missing these critically important teeth. It must take a particularly heartless dentist to remove such a tooth without making every effort to save it. Many years ago Dr. Dodes had just opened his office and a woman brought in her six-year-old son with a painful lower first molar. Dr. D. recommended removing part of the nerve and placing a medicated filling in the tooth. This might allow the roots to complete their growth and the tooth to be saved. The parent refused, and when she saw Dr. D. a few days later, she accused him of being a crook because of the fee he wanted for saving the tooth when Dr. Poorwork was happy to pull the tooth for less.

COMMON PROBLEMS IN CHILDREN'S DENTAL DEVELOPMENT

Occasionally a permanent tooth fails to come in. This can be a serious problem. The usual treatment is to use orthodontics and bonding, or, once the patient is an adult, a fixed bridge or an implant to replace the missing tooth. Sometimes people develop extra teeth. They may be harmless and easily removed, or they may cause serious problems by blocking the growth of another tooth.

Another developmental problem is a deformed permanent tooth. Sometimes this is caused by a badly infected but untreated baby tooth; sometimes no known cause exists. Many of these teeth can be beautifully fixed with a bonded composite (tooth-colored plastic) filling. Now and then, a tooth is so deformed that it has to be extracted and either orthodontics or fixed bridges or implants supplied.

Children accidentally get hit in the mouth all the time, and this kind of trauma often damages the teeth. A front baby tooth may be knocked out years before it was scheduled to be replaced. Treatment is rarely necessary in such a case, since the front teeth do not have the critical space-maintenance functions of the primary molars. The dentist should use X rays to check the developing permanent tooth buds for any damage, but it is very rare that such an injury causes damage.

If a baby front tooth is knocked loose, keep the child on soft foods until it tightens up. If the tooth turns dark, this indicates that there was bleeding into the hollow space called the pulp chamber within the tooth. As a rule, no treatment is necessary, since by the time the dying pulp becomes infected so that it can give trouble, it is time for the tooth to be replaced anyway; baby front teeth are usually lost by the age of seven. Although injuries of this type are common and usually not serious, it's difficult for parents to be casual about them. The child comes home in pain, screaming, with a greatly swollen and bloodied lip; the gum is swollen, purplish-blue, and oozing blood; and the tooth is quite loose and hurts when it's moved. The child, sensing the parents' anxiety, howls even more. Yet as a rule, the pain soon goes away, the swelling goes down in a day or two, and the child forgets about the wound. But as a precaution, see a dentist promptly. (See Chapter 7 for more information on first aid for tooth injuries.)

By far the most common cause of serious trouble is the premature loss of a primary molar, and this factor is, of course, controllable. If a primary first molar is lost, a space-maintaining appliance, either fixed or removable, is advised. But the best way to avoid the premature loss of the primary teeth is by properly caring for the child's teeth. And yet many people, and even some dentists, still believe that baby teeth are unimportant and need not be cared for. This absurd attitude has been encouraged by some dentists who don't want to make the effort or take the time to work on children's teeth. Instead of being responsible and compassionate and sending the child to another dentist who is willing to work on children, they neglect the child's needs. Suffice it to say that a child's teeth deserve the same careful care as do the teeth of an adult, and that failure to provide good care can have irreparable consequences. To that often-asked question, must we bother with children's teeth, there is only one answer, a loud, unequivocal yes!

AVERAGE TOOTH GROWTH

There is great variation in the normal growth of both the primary (baby) teeth and the secondary (permanent) teeth. Don't be upset if your child's teeth don't appear within the time periods shown, which are just rough estimates. If you have questions, ask your dentist. A child should be examined by the age of three at the latest.

Primary centrals and lateral incisors	6–13 months	Permanent centrals and lateral incisors	6–9 years
Primary cuspids	16–23 months	Permanent cuspids and premolars	9–12 years
Primary molars	13–33 months	Permanent first molars	6–8 years
		Permanent second molars	11–13 years
		Permanent third molars (wisdom teeth)	17–21 years

CHILD ABUSE

Child abuse and neglect are significant problems for American society. In 1992 it was estimated that almost three million children were victims of mistreatment (as reported to child protection agencies). To help discover and alleviate child abuse, all the state legislatures have passed laws requiring dentists to report suspected abuse and neglect to the proper authorities. Under these laws, dentists are listed as "mandated reporters" and are legally required, under penalty of law, to report any case in which a child they see is suspected of being abused or neglected. Involving dentists in this way makes sense, since more than 65 percent of all cases of physical abuse involve injuries to the head, neck, or mouth. But less than 1 percent of all reports of abuse are filed by dentists.

In most states dentists are also required to take courses on child abuse detection as part of their continuing education activities. As dentists become more aware of their moral and legal responsibilities, their reporting of abuse cases will increase. With an annual incidence of more than two thousand child abuse fatalities per year, dentists must increase their level of awareness and fulfill their ethical duties in reporting suspected child abusers.

Part III

*

Quackery

19. A Primer on Quackery

*

A GENERATION OF SUCKERS

P. T. Barnum said, "There's a sucker born every minute." If he lived today he might say there's one born every second. Not since before the Pure Food and Drug Act in 1906 have Americans been so credulous, so willing to believe pure nonsense, so willing to be duped. Medical scams, some even with the blessings of the law, abound. Useless "homeopathic" medicines are now sold in many drugstores, despite the fact that the druggists selling them know they are worthless.

Books on these subjects regularly become best-sellers. The media take joy in straight-faced reporting of these lies, giving much less emphasis to the truth. Even Congress gets into the act. Mostly lawyers rather than scientists, many of our elected representatives are partisan to quack notions, and this tendency is greatly reinforced by the political contributions generated by the well-financed quack establishment. One particularly devastating result of the quacks' relentless lobbying of Congress has been the recent passage of amendments to the Dietary Supplement Health and Education Act that removed legal restraints from the labeling and advertising of food "supplements." This consumer disaster has opened the floodgates for fraudulent advertising of quack nostrums. The other day we heard a radio ad claiming that a food supplement medicine strengthened the immune system, got rid of cellulite, reduced weight, and prevented heart attacks and cancer. All in all, the ad made about a dozen medical health claims for the product, none of them proven or even plausible. This ad and others equally phony have been made possible by that shameful action of Congress.

What has made us so gullible that we will throw our money away on useless medicines, phony "cures," and all kinds of quacks and frauds? Is it that the television-driven culture prefers fantasy to reality? Is it that the real world has become so complex and difficult to understand that the retreat to fantasy is easier on our emotional resources? Is it the paranoia of not trusting the conventional experts, such as doctors, and instead placing our faith in the quacks, who appear so much more sympathetic? (We recall with a rueful smile a quack chiropractor who told us, "The most important thing in relating to a patient is sincerity, and as soon as you learn to fake that you've got it made.")

We often hear that alternative health care is popular because of the shortcomings of establishment doctors. Establishment doctors, it is claimed, are arrogant, uncaring, wealthy, and only interested in getting wealthier, while alternative healers take more time with you, are sympathetic, and a lot cheaper.

We disagree with this popular explanation. We feel that conventional health care has become a victim of its own success. Early in the century medicine had little more to offer than the quacks. No one was surprised when sick people were not cured or died. But the discovery of antibiotics and other dramatically potent drugs and spectacular advances in surgical techniques have made modern medicine so successful that the public expects a cure in every case. The doctor, bound by integrity, cannot promise to cure hopeless cases, but the quack can and does. No one likes to hear that his prospects are poor and that treatment is expensive; one prefers to hear that the quack's magic (and usually cheap) methods will prevail. And too many people are falling prey to these deceptions.

Whatever the explanation, we are confronted with the disagreeable fact that pseudoscience is a large, disturbing presence in our contemporary world, and those who learn to recognize and avoid it will save not only their money but also their health and, quite possibly, their lives.

Nor are dentists immune to the pseudoscientific enticement and financial incentives of quackery; many dentists are including these lucrative frauds in their practices. The following sections discuss in detail a variety of medical frauds and quackeries that have been adopted by dentists. It well behooves the reader who doesn't want to become a sucker to read this section carefully.

Russell Baker has characterized those who run American culture as a bunch of frauds, quacks, clowns, montebanks, and imbeciles. Don't be taken in: Don't be another sucker.

THE TOOLS OF THE QUACK

Many well-educated, skeptical people suffer from a failure of logic when it comes to matters of health. Some studies suggest that the more educated the person, the more likely he is to fall for some form of quackery. A major logical failing of the educated, although it is rarely recognized for what it is, is prejudice. Too many believe that everything "natural" is good, that "chemicals" somehow are unhealthful; that "organic" is good and "artificial" is bad. This is prejudice, as illogical as saying that all foreigners are bad. The wise question is not whether something is "natural" or "chemical," "new" or "old," "organic" or "additive," but whether something is *good* or *bad*. Not all chemicals are bad, and not everything natural is good. And all that is original and novel is not necessarily good. "It's easier to be original and foolish than original and wise," said Leibniz. Here are some ways the quack fools most of the people most of the time.

Sometimes people believe in something so fervently that they adjust any contrary information to fit into their already held belief system. The person holding such beliefs and confronted by evidence that he is wrong may react emotionally and consider the evidence to be a personal attack. He will then deny the evidence, no matter how strong it is. This emotional reaction is part of common human nature; it takes a strong, objective mind to combat it, and it is exploited by the quacks.

Evidence, to be acceptable, must follow the rules. Evidence based on logical fallacies, poorly designed or faked studies, and testimonials and anecdotes is not acceptable; these are the methods of quacks. The alternative to evidence is guesswork. We prefer science to pseudoscience, scientifically gathered evidence to the opinions of those who profit by their pronouncements. "Alternative" medicine is a red herring; *there is no alternative to proper treatment*. "Alternative" means another method of similar effectiveness: A train and a bus are transportation alternatives; aspirin, Tylenol, or Advil are reasonable over-the-counter alternatives for pain. But a flying carpet is not an alternative to an airplane, nor is a quack remedy an alternative to proper treatment.

The fallacy of the appeal to authority is another pitfall exploited by the quacks. Credentials can be phony, meaningless, or bought. Even people with genuine credentials can be dead wrong.

Citing credentials or quoting authorities are no guarantees of reliability. Many quacks boast of fancy-sounding degrees from unaccredited mail-order diploma mills and display impressive-looking but meaningless plaques on the wall. A dentist whom we once interviewed had a particularly beautiful and impressive diploma on the wall of his treatment room. It was from a dog obedience school.

WHY PEOPLE BELIEVE QUACKS

Many intelligent people to some extent retain the rebelliousness of youth under the guise of "individuality." They are resentful of authority and the establishment; they may be jealous of "wealthy doctors"; they may harbor the desire to have trendy knowledge ("I'm smarter they they are, I'm up on the latest"). And a touch of paranoia can play its part ("The establishment is trying to conceal the truth about cancer, the environment, nutrition, but they can't fool me. I get my information from courageous and outspoken scientific pioneers."). Quackery can be appealing because it's consistent with the American notion of freedom and individuality and resistance to control and dogma.

It's common for quacks to claim that the medical community is plotting against them, usually for economic reasons. They don't explain why doctors would allow themselves and their families to suffer from diseases that are curable by these "miracle treatments." We've been challenged by some promoters to test products and methods that we've criticized. This is not our responsibility but theirs. The promoter who is going to profit from a treatment has the obligation to test thoroughly and prove safety and efficacy before selling to the public. In a few cases where the product was tested by research scientists and found to be worthless, the promoters then accused the scientists of being biased; they never admitted that their remedy failed. In the late 1970s the promoters of laetrile mounted a successful political campaign to have the National Cancer Institute sponsor a clinical trial comparing laetrile with a placebo. When the study showed that laetrile was useless, its promoters claimed that the trial design had been flawed. Today we have a section of the National Institutes of Health dedicated to studying "alternative therapies." Unfortunately, the person who was initially appointed to oversee this agency resigned because he demanded scientific proof, not just testimonials, before he would allow health claims to be validated by the NIH. The new chief doesn't appear to adhere to the stringent scientific rules. The null hypothesis (one of the central philosophical supports for the scientific method) states: "A treatment or diagnostic test is considered unsafe and ineffective until proved otherwise." Thus the responsibility for proof rests with those advancing a method, treatment, or theory *before* it reaches the marketplace; one should not have to disprove every aberrant product or idea in order to remove it from the marketplace.

Quacks echo the wail of pseudoscience when they say that some day a controlled study will validate their theories. This exactly contradicts the requirements of real scientific medicine—that a treatment be used only *after* scientific proof of its safety and effectiveness has been offered, not in the hope that maybe it will be validated in the future.

Remedies used prior to proof are called experiments, and should be so labeled. The use of unproved treatments represented as legitimate to patients, for money, is a good description of quackery.

QUACKS COUNT ON:

- The placebo effect, which about half the time improves chronic symptoms. The quack is quick to take the credit.

- The waxing and waning of chronic symptoms. When the symptom gets worse, the patient goes to the quack, who takes the credit when the symptom gets cyclically better, as it would have done anyway.

- Misdiagnosis. A favorite quack trick is to tell you you have a disease you don't have, then cure you.

- Spontaneous remission. Occasionally, a serious disease improves or gets better for no detectable reason. The quack loudly takes credit, without mentioning his many failures.

- Phony "prevention" programs. It's very easy to "cure" a patient who has nothing the matter with him. Often the patient is a willing accomplice to the deception (or self-deception).

QUACKERY AND THE LAW

Quackery is not necessarily illegal; in any case, it is very difficult to prosecute even the most flagrant quackery. But the public erroneously believes that it is protected from quackery by the law. This gives a false sense of security and makes it easier for the quack to deceive. The quack is often able to hoodwink scientifically illiterate judges and juries, and then points to the favorable law decision as "proof" of his theories. The quack prefers the courts of law to the courts of science. His chances are much better with the law. The law says: "You are innocent until proved guilty." Science says the opposite: "You are guilty until proved innocent." A treatment shouldn't be used *until it is scientifically proved safe and effective.*

METHODS OF THE QUACK

The quack makes unscientific claims and defies you to disprove them. A real scientist develops and displays proof before making claims; a real doctor has scientific evidence that a treatment is safe and effective before he uses it.

The quack uses complicated language and systems to cover up a simple but nonscientific principle. Many chiropractors claim that all disease stems from misalignments of the spine; the dental TMJ quack claims that numerous diseases come from misalignment of the jaw joint. These are simple (in the sense of "simpleton") concepts that are dressed up in all sorts of complicated pseudolanguage. Additionally, quack jargon commonly makes use of emotionally loaded catchwords ("alternative," "holistic," "prevention," "nutrition," "immune system," "wellness"). Quacks claim to "strengthen" or "bolster the immune system," "detoxify," "purify," or "rejuvenate" your body, "balance your body's chemistry or its energy flow," or "bring you into harmony with nature." William

Lutz calls this "doublespeak," which "perverts the essential function of language, which is communication, in order to mislead, distort, deceive, circumvent."

A striking example of doublespeak is provided by promoters of alternative therapies who describe conventional cancer therapy as "cut, burn, and poison." The real words are, of course, "surgery, radiation, and chemotherapy"—effective treatments that have saved thousands of lives. But the emotionally loaded doublespeak euphemisms of quacks have killed many unsophisticated patients by scaring them away from effective treatment. We offer the wisdom of Confucius: "When words lose their meaning, men lose their liberty."

Quacks claim to know secret cures. Forget about it. Scientists share breakthroughs and publish their results. This is how the Nobel Prize is won—not by keeping a fabulous discovery a secret!

The quack always finds a way to make a profit on his theories. He relies on authoritarianism, logical fallacies, falsehoods, unsupported assertions, anecdotes, and testimonials. He never defends his methods by showing proof but instead attacks the "establishment." He responds to criticism by threatening to sue rather than by demonstrating proof. He always comes up with something "new." As soon as we disprove one thing he is ready with something else, equally fallacious.

If the quack is wrong ninety-nine times and turns out to be right once, the claim is made, pointing to the one time he was right, that the quack is a courageous pioneer.

If the legitimate doctor is right ninety-nine times and wrong once, the quacks loudly point out the one time the establishment was wrong.

The quack promises quick dramatic, painless, miraculous cures. Often these promises are made subtly so that they can be denied later, when the authorities start closing in. Absolute safety is also usually guaranteed, but something that has the power to cure also has the ability to harm, and treatments that have no side effects rarely have the strength to cure.

"QUACK-SENSITIVE" DISEASES

"Quack-sensitive diseases" is the name we give to those ailments that quacks always claim to cure. These are genuine ailments whose diagnosis, causes, and treatments are uncertain and that often are aggravated by emotional components. Examples include arthritis, headaches, chronic nonspecific discomfort, loss of "vigor," general malaise, multiple sclerosis, depression, sexual difficulties, "immune system deficiency," Alzheimer's and Parkinson's diseases. These are ailments characterized by chronic discomfort and which often incorporate emotional factors. Conventional medicine finds these difficult to treat successfully. The quack hurls himself into the breach. The astute reader will realize that these "quack-sensitive" diseases are the same conditions claimed to be cured or prevented by holistic nutritionists, acupuncturists, errant chiropractors, faith healers, TMJ quacks, and dubious healers of every stripe. Patient beware!

THE SINCERE QUACK

If the quack is sincere and really believes in what he's doing, does that make it all right? Perhaps it's safer to go to the quack who knows he is a quack; at least fear of legal reprisal may prevent him from killing you. The sincere quack may kill you in his sincerity, as he has often killed himself and his family. Recently a Long Island chiropractor, thirty-five years old, died in Mexico where his cancer was being treated with the "alternative holistic" methods he believed in. Many dentists who use quack methods sincerely believe in these methods.

CONFUSE THE CONSUMER

"MAY YOU NEVER KNOW WHAT WE'RE PREVENTING!" This statement is from an advertising "newsletter" put out by a so-called holistic dentist. What he is, in essence, saying, "Prevention is good, and what I do constitutes scientific prevention." He pretends that because the first part of his implication is true (prevention is good), then the second part must also be true (what he does constitutes prevention). If challenged, he defends the first half of his implication and condemns you for attacking "prevention," as if his methods and prevention were one and the same. It takes one experienced in critical thinking to see through this ploy.

IGNORING THE PROBLEM

Perhaps most puzzling is the reluctance of legitimate practitioners to go after the quacks. The legitimate doctor may be afraid that criticism of quackery will open the floodgates of criticism to the whole profession. But quackery is on the rise, and if not opposed could deal a serious blow to the ability to practice quality health care. In dentistry, Dr. Goodwork must come to realize that the quack is his competition and has a significant unfair competitive advantage. Why should anyone go to Dr. Goodwork, who can tend only to the teeth and mouth, while he can go to Dr. Quack, who can also cure multiple sclerosis and ensure long-lasting health. The only defense Dr. Goodwork has is to expose to the public the fact that Dr. Quack is a liar, that he cannot cure multiple sclerosis and ensure long-lasting health. We hope that this book will stimulate others to join the fight against quackery and incompetence.

LOGIC AND STATISTICS—COMING TO CONCLUSIONS

Every day we are bombarded with claims, often conflicting, about our health. How can we deal with these claims? Should I have my silver fillings removed to prevent multiple sclerosis? Can my headaches be helped by having my teeth ground down? Must my teeth, which have had root canal treatment, be extracted before they poison my whole body? Some of these questions literally involve life or death: Should I follow my doctor's advice and have my cancer treated with radiation, or should I listen to my guru and go on a macrobiotic diet? Should my heart be treated with the cardiologist's medicine or the naturopath's vitamins?

The wrong answer, the wrong decision could mean wasted

time, thrown-away money, possible lifelong pain and disability, or, in the common enough worst scenario, loss of life itself. What can we believe? When inundated with claims and presented with statistics, is there a preferred method for coming to accurate conclusions?

There is, and it's called scientific method, or critical thinking, or skeptical thinking. We urge every reader to learn how to think scientifically. A complete exposition of the techniques of critical thinking is beyond the scope of this book, but we can offer a few maxims that can serve as a start in the right direction.

Brief Introduction to Critical Thinking

I know he's open minded; I can feel the draft from here.
—Groucho Marx

Most important in critical thinking is the old but sensible caution: Be a skeptic; don't believe everything you hear. It is important to recognize the kinds of medical claims you should *not* believe. Among these are what logicians call unsupported assertions: anecdotes and testimonials.

An anecdote is a story, perhaps told by a doctor, about the result of a treatment: "My patient was unable to conceive, but since I ground down her teeth, she has had two children." A testimonial is a claim, usually made by a patient: "I couldn't have a child, but since my fillings were removed I've had two children."

It is crucial to recognize anecdotes and testimonials and more crucial not to *take them at face value*. Anecdotes and testimonials have no place in scientific reasoning. (The astute reader will recognize that most TV ads are nothing but anecdotes or testimonials, a commentary on their validity.)

When we talk about unsupported assertions, the next question is: What is support? Or better, What is legitimate support? This leads to the greatest difficulties in scientific thinking. Support means evidence, and what constitutes valid evidence is the subject of profound study, involving statistics, experimental protocols, and expert evaluations. A reader glancing at one of the studies printed in a respected scientific journal, the *New England Journal of Medicine (NEJM),* for example, will be amazed at the extreme care taken in the design and execution of the experiments reported. This care is necessary to minimize sources of error. Although even the *NEJM* has been fooled, it is generally safe to consider what is written in such a journal to be reliable. Newspaper accounts, even newspaper accounts of scientific articles, are much less reliable. Although many of these news stories are accurate, many of them aren't. Reporters often do not understand scientific thinking and draw unwarranted conclusions from scientific reports.

We should mention that an unsupported assertion is not necessarily false, but it should raise your skeptical vigilance. Judgment and experience come into play here. For example, if your spouse says, "I mailed the mortgage payment," that is an unsupported assertion that has a high probability of being true. Other unsupported assertions may be less reliable, for example, "The check is in the mail."

Statistics and Scientific Reasoning

As Mark Twain said, "There are three kinds of lies: lies, damned lies, and statistics." Or, as another wag put it, "Figures can't lie, but liars can figure."

The noted mathematician Dr. John Allen Paulos has pointed out in his fascinating books on "innumeracy" that most of us are

---

Gynecological Problems Are Serious Illnesses

DEAR WOMEN,

Your doctor should know that a 98% correlation exists between women who have menstrual problems (excessive bloating, cramping and/or bleeding) and women who also have TMJ problems.

One of the most common logical errors is the confusion between correlation and causation. In this ad, from one of our community newspapers, the dentist doesn't seem to realize that there is a 100 percent correlation between woman who have menstrual problems and women who talk on the telephone. But one doesn't *cause* the other. This may seem comical but not to the woman with a serious gynecological problem.

bewildered by the magnitude of numbers and are likely to misinterpret coincidence as cause and effect. An example is the recent fear of cellular phones. When a person who uses a cellular phone is found to have brain cancer, the phone is immediately accused of being the cause. Yet the public is uninterested in or doesn't understand the important statistical data that exonerates cell phones. Statisticians can determine what percentage of people who don't use a cellular phone get brain cancer. They have found that seven of every hundred thousand Americans get brain cancer each year. Cell phone users do not have a higher incidence of brain cancer and therefore, the statistical evidence is that the two occurrences, cell phone use and cancer, are not related; it is a coincidence. In all the news stories we've seen on this topic, the essential statistics have never been stated or explained. Thus many Americans, to this day, erroneously believe that cell phone use is linked to brain cancer.

Lies and Damned Lies

Statistics and numbers are easy to ignore or misinterpret, and Mark Twain's observation becomes a sobering truth when we consider reactions to pesticides, fluoride, tobacco, alcohol, and illegal substances. Tobacco, by far our greatest health threat, leads to 400,000 deaths annually, a total that dwarfs alcohol's 90,000 deaths. Yet we seem to be far more concerned with illegal drugs, which account for "only" 20,000 annual deaths.

Similarly, some residents of Long Island are very concerned about pesticide residues, and the water supply in Nassau County is not fluoridated because of fears of "chemicals." However, nature provides an enormous amount of naturally occurring pesticides that plants have evolved to protect themselves against insects and microorganisms, and these chemicals are every bit as toxic as artificial pesticides. Bruce Ames, a respected biochemist, has estimated that we eat ten thousand times as much natural pesticide (hydrazines in mushrooms, aflatoxins in peanuts, etc.) as we do man-made additives, but most people are not aware of this, mistakingly thinking that "natural" pesticides are not toxic. This misunderstanding of statistics leads to the substitution of prejudice for reasoning, the prejudice lying in the assumption that "natural" substances are okay, while "chemical" artificial substances must be harmful.

Probability

Statistical quacks often try to prove their point by citing results of studies that seemingly defy the laws of probability. "The chance of our experimental result happening under ordinary circumstances is less than five thousand to one, so what we were doing must have caused this improbable result." Such statements are often heard to substantiate quack claims about ESP, psychic healing, or other odd-ball techniques. But the 5,000-to-1 odds are taken out of context. As an example, consider a golfer about to hit a ball to the fairway. The fairway contains billions of blades of grass, and the ball lands on one of them. It was indeed a billion to one against the ball landing on that particular blade of grass, but is it reasonable to claim that something spectacular has happened? The ball had to land somewhere, and anywhere it landed would have been a billion-to-one shot.

Statistics fakers love to take their numbers out of context. One toothpaste advertisement claimed something like "37 percent less cavities with our new formula." But 37 percent less than *what?* The research that backed up this claim was flawed by uncontrolled variables as well as being out of context.

Here is an example of a common out-of-context error: confusing a rate of increase with the total picture. Two twelve-year-old boys are exactly five feet tall. Six months later, one of these boys has grown three-quarters of an inch, and the other boy has grown a half inch: one is now five feet and three-quarters of an inch tall, while the other boy is five feet and one-half inch tall. When the boys stand next to each other they look exactly the same height. However, in that six-month period, one boy has grown 50 percent more than the other boy! (Three-quarters of an inch is 50 percent more than half an inch.) Now, 50 percent is an impressive number, unless you take the measurements in context. If you consider the *total* picture, the total height of the boys, one child is now 0.41 percent taller than the other, a hundredfold difference from 50 percent.

For those stalwart readers who plowed through the numbers

in those examples it should be clear why the contemplation of statistics both fascinates and repels us. The advantage of proper interpretation of these data is obvious: a better and deeper understanding of the world in which we live. The misunderstanding of the rules of critical thinking can lead to the false indictment of entire industries and dangerously incorrect medical conclusions.

20. Quackery in Dentistry

*

Many of the topics covered in this chapter are claimed by some to be controversial. We remind you that a controversy is a disputation concerning matters of *opinion*. Once opinion is replaced by *fact,* controversy disappears. Quacks like to call their assertions "controversial." They are not controversial; they are merely wrong.

Quackery, the promotion of false or unproven medical schemes for profit, has a long history, but it is relatively new to dentistry. A number of factors, mostly adding up to an economic squeeze on dentists, have made some dentists willing to consider quackery.

Quackery has always had popular appeal, because the outrageous health promises of the quack are attractive to the public, and this gives the quack a substantial and monumentally unfair competitive advantage over the legitimate practitioner. And quackery is easy; the only skill it requires is the ability to look a fellow human being in the eye, lie to him, and take his money. Fortunately, many of us are by nature and background unable to develop this skill.

Experts on dental health fraud estimate that more than $3 billion a year is wasted on quack dentistry. The problem has received some serious attention in such publications as the *Journal of the American Dental Association.* But no effective action has been taken to combat the quacks. The following sections will acquaint you with areas of unproven or disproven dental treatments. Very few dentists have adopted all these techniques; dental quacks usually pick and choose, a little of this and a little of that. Judging from the popularity of quack dental courses, we believe your chance of using a dentist who has adopted some of these quack techniques is fairly high. Many dentists have seen a decrease in patients and more openings in their daily schedules, and for some of them quackery has been an easy and lucrative way out. Since organized dentistry has not taken effective steps to control dental quackery, we hope that our efforts to educate the public about quackery will result in fewer patients getting victimized.

A NOTE ON CREDENTIALS

All of us are generally impressed by credentials. But, as we noted previously, credentials are an area of possible fraud and deception.

A dental degree requires a minimum of two years of undergraduate college followed by four years of dental school. However, almost all students entering dental school have graduated from four-year colleges. After graduating from dental school, national and state or regional board exams must be passed before a dentist is licensed to practice. There are more than 145,000 licensed dentists in the United States. They hold either a Doctor of Dental Surgery (DDS) degree or the equivalent Doctor of Medical Dentistry (DMD) degree.

WHAT YOU SHOULD KNOW ABOUT SPECIALISTS

The American Dental Association recognizes eight specialties. A board-qualified dental specialist must have at least two years of advanced training, accredited by the ADA Council on Dental Education, after graduating from dental school. The specialist is required to limit his practice to the area of specialization. The eight genuine areas of specialization are:

1. Endodontics (root canal): diagnosis and treatment of diseases of the pulp (nerve) and related structures
2. Oral pathology: diagnosis of tumors, other diseases, and injuries of the head and neck
3. Oral and maxillofacial surgery: tooth extractions; diagnosis and surgical treatment of diseases, injuries, and defects of the mouth, jaw and face
4. Orthodontics: diagnosis and correction of tooth alignment and facial deformities
5. Pediatric dentistry: dental care of infants and children
6. Periodontics: diagnosis and treatment of diseases of the gums and related structures

7. Prosthodontics: diagnosis and treatment involving the replacement of missing teeth
8. Public health dentistry: prevention and control of dental disease and promotion of community dental health

Some dentists who have not completed the training required by the ADA but who limit their practice or emphasize one area of treatment refer to themselves as specialists. Many such dentists practice in a scientific and ethical manner, doing high-quality work. However, some dentists claim to be specialists in fields that are either unrecognized, unscientific, or both. The public's problem of recognizing quackery is made difficult by the easy availability of meaningless but impressive and confusing credentials. There are a number of unaccredited diploma mills operating in the United States which, for a fee, will provide a variety of phony credentials. Quacks often claim membership in impressive-sounding but bogus or unrecognized professional organizations. Anyone claiming to be a certified dental "specialist" who does not limit his practice and it not certified in one of the recognized dental specialties is being fraudulent. Examples of areas that are *not* dental specialties include: "cosmetic dentistry," "TMJ," "holistics," "bonding," "nonsurgical periodontics," "nutrition," "prevention," "amalgam detoxification," and "kinesiology."

A few phonies claim they are specialists based on their viewing of a short videotape or attendance at a weekend seminar, and they point to a nicely laminated plaque on the wall as substantiation. Remember, phony credentials can be bought and easily faked. Consumers must be wary of bogus degrees (particularly in "nutrition") from unaccredited correspondence schools, membership certificates from organizations with impressive-sounding names but no scientific standing, and "diplomas" that are often distributed at so-called continuing education courses. Although most continuing education courses are valid, unscientific theories and practices are taught at far too many of them.

HOLISTIC DENTISTRY

Many dental charlatans call themselves "holistic." "Holistic" is a legitimate word that properly means to consider every available appropriate treatment for the whole patient, including attention to emotional factors, lifestyle, and prevention. But the quack has subverted this word to mean every and any treatment, however inappropriate, for which he can get a fee. Holistic dental offices seem to be more interested in medical than dental procedures, and health claims made by holistic dentists seem clearly beyond the boundaries or competence of dental practice.

Prevention is an important goal of health care, especially in dentistry, where good dentists understand how to prevent or control most major dental disease. But prevention is an area much abused by quacks. In the dental office these phony prevention schemes usually involve the purchase of expensive nutritional supplements or a plastic bite appliance. A common quack claim is that unique methods known to the quack can prevent disease and maintain "optimum" health, or, as the "holistic" quack so often puts it, "promote wellness." These evasive words have no scientific meaning. "Wellness" is not even in our dictionaries; the real word is *health*. Judging from the use of the word in quack literature, wellness is the disease quacks treat when there is nothing wrong with the patient. And these treatments are remarkably successful; it's easy to cure patients who aren't sick.

The Academy of General Dentistry, the second largest group of American dentists, has estimated that at least 5 percent of dentists consider themselves "holistic." As for the potential hazards to patients, "holistic" dentistry can lead not only to wasting money but also to misdiagnosis, treatment for a nonexistent disease, or improper treatment for a serious and potentially life-threatening disorder.

THE ANTIFLUORIDATION MOVEMENT

The antifluoridation movement uses typical quack arguments and tactics. Whenever one phony claim is disproved, they come up with another. It has been said, and we firmly believe, that every child living in a *non*fluoridated area is a victim of quackery.

Fluoride, one of the most abundant elements on Earth, is a mineral found naturally in many water supplies. Low dosages of ingested fluoride cause developing teeth to greatly increase their resistance to decay. Fluoride also reduces decay when applied topically to teeth.

In 1945 the first controlled fluoridation program in the United States was begun in Grand Rapids, Michigan. Today more than 135 million people in the United States drink water that is fluoridated, either artificially or naturally. In the late 1960s the World Health Organization pulled together most of the known research on fluoride in order to provide an impartial review. They evaluated worldwide population studies, experimental research, animal studies, and clinical investigations including human autopsy studies, clinical trials, and X-ray research. The report, "Fluorides and Human Health," was published in 1970 and concluded that there was no reliable evidence that any ill effects or symptoms result from drinking water that is fluoridated at recommended levels. In addition, fluoride is probably the cheapest public health measure ever found. It costs about 50¢ per person per year, and it saves an estimated $80 per person in yearly dental treatment costs.

Last summer a mother brought in her three-year-old daughter for examination. The child's mouth was ridden with decay. We checked for the usual suspects: bottle with milk or juice at night, excess candy consumption, poor diet, poor oral hygiene. The mother said no to each of these. We asked where the child was born and where they lived, suspecting it was an area without fluoride, but she did indeed come from a fluoridated area. We told the mother that the reason for the child's condition was hard to understand and that we hadn't seen such a damaged mouth in a youngster since before the days of fluoride, when such situations were common. "Our family is very health conscious," she replied, "and we drink only bottled water!"

Despite the scientific evidence and the success of fluoridation, a vociferous minority has risen in opposition. Made up mostly of food faddists, cultists, chiropractors, and people who misunderstand what fluoridation is, the antifluoridation movement has succeeded in having fluoride removed from some water systems and not installed in others. The efforts of the antifluoridationists have also been aided by certain fringe physicians, dentists, and scientists, and those citizens who don't believe that government has a proper function in pursuing public health. Some of the funding for the antifluoridation movement is provided by supplement and health food manufacterers who sell useless products, usually containing calcium, with the claims that they will prevent decay "naturally" and that fluoride (which, in reality, is their competition) is dangerous and not needed.

In 1990 an article in *Newsweek* suggested that fluoridation is ineffective and dangerous. The article was the result of a misunderstanding of the unintended release of preliminary data from an experiment at the National Institute of Environmental Health Sciences, in which rats and mice were exposed to very high doses of fluoride. A few of the animals developed bone cancer, but a thorough review of the study by the U.S. Public Health Service concluded that the data were insignificant and that fluoridation posed no risk of causing cancer or any other disease.

Fluoridation is the most thoroughly studied scientific program in all history. Entire populations have been used in controlled studies. The substance of all this research has been neatly summarized by Consumers Union: "The simple truth is that there's no 'scientific controversy' over the safety of fluoridation. The practice is safe, economical, and beneficial. The survival of this fake controversy represents one of the major triumphs of quackery over science in our generation."

TEMPOROMANDIBULAR JOINT DISORDERS (TMJ)

TMJ, a "disease" unheard of a generation ago, now seems to be reaching epidemic proportions. In some dental offices every patient walking in is diagnosed as having TMJ. Books can be written on the TMJ scam alone, which has been described as dentistry's "hottest" area of unorthodoxy and out-and-out quackery.

TMJ properly stands for temporomandibular joint, the neuromuscular hinge connecting the movable lower jaw to the skull (the upper jaw is connected to the skull and is not movable). TMJ has come to be used to describe a confusing and nonspecific muddle of conditions and symptoms, all allegedly caused by a malfunction of the TM joint. But the joint is rarely the cause of these symptoms, so many prefer the name TMD (temporomandibular disorders). The most common symptom of TMD is chronic facial pain, fairly constant pain of more than three months' duration. This pain is usually accompanied by difficulty in moving the lower jaw.

TMJ quacks make the scientifically unsupported claim that a "bad bite" causes a wide variety of symptoms including headaches, facial pain, muscular weakness, fatigue, menstrual cramps, scoliosis, general discomfort, and even athletic and sexual difficulties. Sound familiar? (Once again we meet the quack-sensitive diseases.)

Most TMD quackery is based on the long-discredited "bad bite" theory, the notion that the TM joint is stressed because the teeth can't come together "properly." Treatment therefore consists in "correcting" the bite by grinding the teeth, or by building up the teeth with dental restorations, or by the use of an invasive "bite-correcting" plastic appliance. These treatments, easy, popular, and lucrative for the quack, are neither safe nor effective for most of the conditions diagnosed as TMD. One of the most popular treatments, the plastic bite-altering appliance (presumptuously called the *m*andibular *o*rthopedic *r*epositioning *a*ppliance, or MORA), can function effectively as a placebo, but it also can make symptoms worse and often causes enough deforming tooth movement to require corrective orthodontic treatment. If a placebo is to be used, it is better to use a noninvasive one such as a flat-plane plastic appliance, and only for limited amounts of time and never while eating.

MORAs should not be confused with night guards, which cover all the teeth and are used to prevent abnormal wearing down of the enamel in people who grind their teeth while sleeping. Sometimes appliances called bite splints, which are similar to night guards, are prescribed to relieve muscle strain in patients with TMJ. Although there is no strong scientific support for the use of bite splints, when properly constructed and used they do not cause any harm or cause movement of the teeth.

There are several surgical treatments for TM disorders, but the failure rate is high, often leaving the patient in continual intractable pain. Surgery should be considered only as a measure of last resort, when a condition amenable to surgery has been definitely diagnosed.

TMD quacks abuse expensive X rays for diagnosis. Jaw joint X rays or MRIs are appropriate when there has been trauma or a history of progressive joint disease, but they should not be taken as a routine screening procedure.

Questionable electronic instruments are gaining popularity for the diagnosis and treatment of alleged TM disorders. These in-

clude surface electromyography, jaw tracking, silent period dura-
tions, electrovibratography, TENS, thermography, sonography,
and Doppler ultrasound. Elaborate and impressive-looking though
they be, none of these devices has been found to be effective for
TMJ treatment or diagnosis. One of the problems with these devices is that they give a high number of false-positive readings,
which means that many patients without disease are diagnosed as
being afflicted with TMD, leading to unnecessary, expensive, and
potentially dangerous treatments. Tests that give a high number of
false-positive results are perfect for the charlatan because he gets a
high rate of success with patients who don't have any disease to
begin with! The most common electronic treatment device is
TENS (transcutaneous electrical nerve stimulation) in which a low-
voltage, low-amperage current is applied to painful body areas.
However, TENS has been found to be no more effective than
placebo therapies. TENS is not dangerous, but it can be quite an
expensive, if futile, treatment. In our office we have a 1902 version
of a TENS machine on display. In the 1800s electricity was promoted as a cure for every known disease, and "medical battery"
devices were very popular. Physicians used them, and they could
be purchased by the public through the Sears catalog. But their effectiveness has not increased since a century ago.

In 1996, the American Association of Electrodiagnostic Medicine (AAEM) published an assessment of surface electomyography
that concluded that "there is no clinical indication for the use of
surface electromyography in the diagnosis and treatment of disorders of nerve or muscle."

TM joint noises (clicking or grinding sounds), even in the
complete absence of symptoms, are often used to make a false
diagnosis. Even when the joint sounds are accompanied by other
symptoms, the noises themselves are not well understood. Often
the joints sounds disappear and the symptoms remain, or the
symptoms disappear and the sounds remain. Joint sounds without
pain or dysfunction do not indicate a disease process and should
not be treated.

A major problem with TMD is that it is imprecisely defined and
poorly understood, even by dentists and physicians. Many physicians, particularly ear, nose, and throat specialists, have been dealing with patients with facial pain they could not diagnose by
sending them to "TMJ specialists" (remember, there is no such rec-

ognized specialty). This plays into the hands of the quacks, who usually start the patient on the familiar round of unscientific and not-needed TMJ appliances and treatments.

Worse yet is the collusion of self-styled TMJ experts with attorneys. Some "TMJ specialists" have been asking attorneys for referrals of accident patients. The TMJ dentists offer to certify the accident victim as having TMJ disorder; this will increase the court-awarded damages for the victim, increase the lawyer's compensation, and, of course, provide a new patient for the TMJ quack.

Courses are being given to dentists and to attorneys in the newly invented nonexistent disease "TMJ whiplash." Mandibular whiplash is a popular diagnosis, usually applied to anyone with an insurance company, an accident (no matter how minor), a lawyer, a crooked dentist, and a jaw joint. In many cases a diagnosis is made only after the patient is introduced to the lawyer, which could be months or even years after the accident. The whiplash-treating dentist will claim that the pain in other injured areas overshadowed and thereby concealed the jaw pain. This flies in the face of everything we know about biology, pain, inflammation, and the joints. If you went jogging and twisted your ankle, the pain would begin at once. You would then rest your leg and, typically, in about a week would be able to use your ankle normally. In common alleged mandibular whiplash cases, the patient is able to use his injured jaw joints for long periods of time before symptoms appear. It's as if you could play basketball with your injured ankle and not notice it. To complicate this scenario, the patient suffering from mandibular whiplash doesn't even need a direct injury to the face. Again, using the ankle analogy: You get hit in the back but your ankle gets injured. As hard as this bogus theory is to believe, many judges have found in favor of dentists suing to receive reimbursement for phony, unnecessary treatments on patients they diagnosed as having mandibular whiplash.

Too many dubious TMJ-related claims have been flooding insurance carriers. Claims for fees in five figures are received for simple electronic gadget or oral appliance treatments that have no scientific basis, and when insurance carriers balk at paying for these fraudulent procedures, the quacks use the courts to force compliance (as we have noted, quacks always look to the courts of law rather than the "courts" of science for support). These abuses decrease insurance capital reserves and result in higher insurance premiums and reduced dental coverage for legitimate procedures.

Even if the court rules in the insurer's favor, the costs of defending the suit are considerable. So insurers tend to negotiate a settlement without a fight, reasoning that it will be cheaper than contesting it in court and facing not only the costs of the action but also the possibility of an adverse judgment. This is because charismatic fakers can run rings around most judges and juries. This melancholy situation will persist until the courts wake up and adopt scientific consensus as a standard for judging health issues.

There is overwhelming evidence that the myriad symptoms usually diagnosed as TMJ respond favorably to simple, inexpensive, and noninvasive treatment. Simple exercises, warm compresses, soft diet, and over-the-counter anti-imflammatory drugs resolve most complaints. Only in a small percentage of cases is additional treatment required. We strongly recommend against invasive, irreversible treatments, and if such treatments are proposed we advise you get a second or even third opinion.

A note is in order on TMJ "specialists." While too many self-styled "TMJ specialists" are indeed quacks, there are legitimate practitioners who focus on facial pain and utilize scientific methods. Not every TMJ doctor is a quack.

A panel convened by the National Institutes of Health concluded on May 1, 1996, after intensive and highly emotional meetings, that there is little scientific evidence for current diagnostic and treatment procedures of TM disorders. "For the majority of TMD patients, the absence of clear guidelines for diagnosis and full range of treatment means that many patients and practitioners may attempt therapy with new and inadequately tested approaches." The panel suggested that there was "overuse of some of the more aggressive treatments" and recommended a conservative and reversible approach for most TMD patients.

One of the most loathsome chapters in the history of American dentistry involved the insertion of a Teflon-coated (Proplast) artifical jaw replacement joint in more than twenty thousand TMJ patients. Although the safety of Teflon in a high-stress bearing area (such as the human jaw) was unknown, the Vitek company got their Teflon-coated implant, the "Proplast jaw joint," past the FDA and vigorously marketed it to maxillofacial surgeons. A maxillofacial surgeon who received a royalty on each implant sold actively promoted the Vitek implant to his colleagues.

In 1984 the first reports of damage from Proplast implants appeared. In 1988 the manufacture and placement of these implants were finally stopped, but that was too late for thousands of people who will require numerous operations to remove and attempt to repair the damage from the Proplast jaw implant. And for many of these patients the damage is uncorrectable and the pain permanent. This would never have happened had the dentists who placed these implants demanded scientific proof that Proplast worked.

HOLISTIC NUTRITION

Traditionally, the only nutrition counseling a dentist provided was advice to avoid sugary foods and snacks. Today "holistic" dentists are promoting a wide variety of food and diet faddism that leads only to swollen profits for the quack. An article by a dentist in a dental trade journal put it most candidly: "Are you interested in doubling your net practice income? We almost did it last year . . . we used nutritional counseling as the vehicle." Of course, "counseling" is a euphemism for selling to trusting patients unneeded and possibly harmful vitamin and food supplements at outrageous markups. Peculiar and discredited diagnostic methods—the lingual ascorbic acid test, hair analysis, cytotoxic testing, and kinesiologic testing—are used to persuade patients to purchase these expensive supplements.

The *Journal of the American Dental Association* has listed the following as examples of unscientific nutrition practice: megavitamin therapy, herbal and oriental medicine, macrobiotic therapy, and even unnecessary vitamin intake. Some dentists are distributors for multilevel companies that market supplements and herbal preparations with suggestions that everyone should use them. Be aware that although nutrition is important in all aspects of health, the promoting of specific for-profit product lines is almost always grounded in greed, not need.

The 1994 Dietary Supplement Health and Education Act seriously weakened the FDA's control over so-called health foods. Sponsored by Senator Orrin Hatch of Utah, the home of many supplement manufacturers, and Representative Bill Richardson of New Mexico, this law allows products with no known food value to be called "food supplements" and permits health claims on their labels and advertising without offering proof or getting prior approval by the FDA. Previously it was required to prove that a product is safe and effective; now, anything goes.

Already the consequences of this act are becoming apparent. There is mounting documentation of crushing side effects, including death, from the unregulated sale of "natural" herbal products containing powerful drugs. People are using these products to get a legal high. Ephedrine, called "speed" by a generation of teenagers, is a major ingredient in many of these so-called food supplements. The FDA has compiled reports on some four hundred "adverse events," including at least fifteen deaths, from ephedrine-containing products. Dr. David Kessler, director of the FDA, says that since the new legislation "we have to be able to prove in court each time that a particular formulation is unsafe if taken as directed. You are always chasing harm after it has occurred. What companies do is reformulate, and we have to start all over again, and because there are many different products and many different combinations, you end up chasing forever."

One wonders about the values of a society where one can go into a "health food" store, make a legal purchase, and get high. Or perhaps die. But, in this enlightened age, what is more important: the public safety, or the profits of the campaign contributors to some senators?

Here are some things to watch out for when evaluating claims about nutrition:

> *Faulty Nutrition.* Ignore any practitioner who claims that most or all diseases are caused by faulty nutrition. Although some diseases are indeed related to diet, most are not. More important, in those cases where diet is a factor, the solution usually is to alter and correct the diet rather than take food supplements and vitamins.
>
> *Poor Nutrition.* Don't believe anyone who tells you most Americans are poorly nourished. Our major illnesses (heart disease and lung cancer) are due to overindulgence, not to deficiency. Life expectancy is advancing, despite our alleged "poor" nutrition. In 1900 the average life expectancy was forty-seven

years of age. Today we can expect to live to nearly eighty. Obviously we are not being poisoned by our food supply.

"Lost" Nutrition. Don't believe anyone who claims that modern food-processing and storage methods remove all the nutritive value from food. Although food processing can change a food's nutrient content, some nutrients will be depleted and others increased. All in all, the changes are not drastic enough to render processed foods worthless. And many foods such as flour and rice are "enriched" to replace nutrients lost in processing.

Single Tests. Don't trust anyone who claims that a single test can be used to determine the body's overall nutritional status. Popular quack diagnostic tests include hair analysis, applied kinesiology, amino acid analysis, cytotoxic testing, live-cell analysis, and herbal crystallization analysis. If any of your health-care providers is using one of these techniques, get another provider.

SILVER-AMALGAM MERCURY "TOXICITY"

Silver amalgam is an alloy of silver, mercury, copper, tin, and zinc. It has been used as a dental filling material for a century and a half and still is the filling of choice for back teeth. Billions of amalgam fillings have been used successfully, with fewer than fifty cases of allergy reported in the literature since 1905. All major health organizations recognize the safety of silver-amalgam fillings, but a group of dentists (often of the "holistic" fringe) are blaming a huge variety of diseases on mercury, which allegedly "leaks" from these fillings into the mouth. The diseases mentioned are the usual quack suspects: multiple sclerosis, immune deficiency diseases, Parkinson's, general malaise, and emotional conditions, among many others (the "quack-sensitive" diseases). The treatment offered by the quacks is the removal of silver fillings and their replacement, usually with plastic, an expensive and traumatic procedure often botched by the quack. This treatment is ironic, since plastic fillings are not as good as silver amalgam and, although generally safe, are still more potentially toxic than amalgam.

Anti-amalgam quacks use typically dubious diagnostic methods; one such device is the "amalgameter." This electronic device (essentially a voltmeter) is claimed to reveal the presence of positively or negatively charged fillings. Some quacks claim that silver fillings must be removed in order of their polarity. This peculiar recommendation is particularly puzzling, since changing the random placement of the leads of such a device can reverse the measured "polarity." The Federal Drug Administration forced the dentist who manufactured these devices to stop production, but many of these and similar phony devices are still in use.

The Jerome mercury tester is a legitimate device that has been used incorrectly by the quacks to diagnose mercury contamination in the mouth. The Jerome analyzer is designed to measure mercury levels in large buildings and giant factory rooms. Its use in the mouth is unreliable. Reliable physiological measurements (blood and urine levels) show that the amount of mercury leaking from these fillings is insignificant. Indeed, if silver fillings did leak mercury in the amounts claimed by the quacks, they would quickly disintegrate. We routinely see silver-amalgam fillings that after half a century are still solid and functioning perfectly.

Quacks and environmental alarmists are quick to inform the public about the toxic substances that surround us. They neglect to mention one of the foundation stones of pharmacology (the study of drugs): Only the dose makes a poison. It makes sense; many of the things we eat or breathe can be dangerous in large doses but are essential at the proper dose. Take table salt. Too much salt can kill you, but without salt we could not live at all. And peaches contain tiny amounts of cyanide. The mercury that may leak out of fillings has a very low level of toxicity, it's not well absorbed through the digestive tract, and there are hundreds of cases of having mercury injected directly into the bloodstream (because of broken rectal thermometers) without any deleterious effects. A person would have to inhale far more mercury than a mouthful of silver-amalgam fillings is capable of releasing, for a very long time, to get any side effects at all.

Perhaps the most compelling evidence refuting the claims of the anti-amalgamists is the fact that American dentists show three to fifteen times the amount of mercury in blood and urine than do the general population, but have no higher incidence of disease, and, in fact, as a group enjoy somewhat better health than the population at large.

The attempt to remove and replace a mouthful of silver fillings can be disastrous to a patient's dental health. A California woman was awarded a substantial settlement from her dentist, who removed her amalgam fillings (claiming they were a "liability" to her large intestine!). As a result, two teeth were lost and two others needed root canal and expensive restoration. And according to *Consumer Reports,* a dentist in Iowa lost his license for five years because he advised a patient with multiple sclerosis to have her amalgams replaced. She was unable to afford his $9,000 fee, so she had all her teeth extracted and replaced with dentures. A month later her MS worsened and she ended up in a hospital. We have seen patients who have been similarly mistreated and are sure that there are multitudes that have gone undocumented; patients of quacks, no matter how abused, are generally reluctant to sue.

The anti-amalgamists have succeeded in getting a flood of media publicity, especially the notorious *60 Minutes* TV segment which was described by famed consumer advocate Dr. Stephen Barrett as "the most irresponsible program ever aired on a health topic." This program sent thousands of people into the hands of quacks, and although the assertions it made have been disproved, *60 Minutes* has never broadcast a retraction. And legislation has actually been introduced (but not passed) in several state legislatures to ban the use of amalgam. This shows, once again, that reporters and lawmakers can be hoodwinked as easily as the rest of us.

And it seems to never end. In February 1996, WABC-TV's *Eyewitness News* broadcast two segments repeating the same tired and discredited claims against amalgam. A couple of British dentists were featured. The accent was different, but the baloney was the same.

Dr. Hal Huggins, a dentist in Colorado, is perhaps the best-known and most outspoken opponent of silver-amalgam fillings. He started taking out amalgams to treat systemic diseases in the 1970s and published a book detailing his theories in 1985. For years Huggins has traveled the world promoting his allegations and teaching dentists, physicians, and others how to diagnose and treat "mercury toxicity." In 1995 a patient of Huggins was awarded $159,000 because he had told her she had to have her fillings removed to preserve her health, which was perfect at that time. She eventually ended up having five teeth pulled, and the replacement bridges Huggins constructed soon fell out.

At the same time the attorney general of Colorado had begun his own investigation into Huggins. At the end of a three-month case, in 1996 the judge recommended that the state revoke Huggins's license. She wrote that Huggins "has taken advantage of the hopes of his patients for an easy fix to their medical problems and has used this to develop a lucrative business for himself. The diagnostic techniques and treatments offered by him at the Huggins Center are scientifically unsupported, without clinical justification and outside the practice of dentistry."

If your dentist tells you that silver fillings are poisonous, find another dentist!

BAKING SODA AND PEROXIDE PERIODONTAL THERAPY

In the late 1970s an oral hygiene program known as the Keyes Technique was widely promoted as a nonsurgical alternative to the accepted surgical methods of treating advanced periodontal disease. The technique involves microscopic examination of the plaque, cleaning the teeth and gums with a mixture of baking soda and peroxide, and treatment with antibiotics. Although there was inadequate research to validate the use of this technique, it became extremely popular with patients, who were all too happy to avoid gum surgery. It was also popular with business-oriented dentists, who found it easy, lucrative, and an excellent marketing tool.

Researchers at the University of Minnesota conducted a four-year controlled study of patients with moderate periodontal disease. The study concluded that although the baking soda mixture did help in maintaining oral health, it was no more effective than ordinary toothpaste. Further, they determined that those using the baking soda regimen were three times more likely to stop their program because it was inconvenient. An FDA panel recently found no convincing evidence that baking soda was effective against gum disease. Baking soda and peroxide therapy has been called "supervised neglect" by a number of experts. It is not needed for moderate problems and allows more serious problems to advance while it masks the symptoms. Dr. Poorwork loves this technique, since it requires no time and no skill to sell a mouthwash to a patient instead of the painstaking and time-consuming scalings required for the correct prevention and treatment of moderate periodontal disease. And it is most attractive to the patient who is told that the deep scaling or surgery won't be needed and that the magic mouthwash will suffice.

QUESTIONABLE PRODUCTS TO FIGHT PERIODONTAL DISEASE

The public is flooded with products to treat periodontal disease and its euphemisms ("bad breath, "gingivitis," "pink toothbrush," etc.). Suffice it to say that there are no over-the-counter magic mouthwashes or toothpastes that are by themselves effective to treat gum disease. The only effective ingredient in toothpaste is fluoride; the rest are useless or possibly harmful. (See Chapter 17.)

A product called AP-24 was recently introduced into the marketplace by the Nu-Skin company of Utah. The active, patented ingredient, called "microdent," is advertised as being effective for the treatment and prevention of periodontal disease. "Microdent" is actually a mixture of silicone lubricants and is being marketed as a huge profit maker for dentists. According to the ADA, independent distributors of AP-24 "are making claims that the product is ADA accepted, FDA approved and that the products control gingivitis and periodontitis. None of these claims is true. . . ."

Oxyfresh is a product sold through a multilevel marketing program and claims to eliminate mouth odors, clean teeth, and "condition" gums. "In the last five years many dentists have built an annual six figure income with a part-time effort," states a dentist-directed ad for Oxyfresh. The active ingredient is chlorine dioxide, which is also used as an algacide in swimming pools. To date there have been no scientifically accepted studies proving any of these claims.

The danger of quack periodontal treatments is that they give patients a false sense of security and cause them to defer effective treatment until it may be too late.

PASTE-FILLER (SARGENTI) ROOT CANAL THERAPY

The root canal is the hollow space within the tooth that contains the tooth's nerve and blood vessels (called the pulp). In case of severe decay or injury, when the pulp becomes damaged or infected, root canal therapy is usually able to save the tooth by removing the infected pulp and filling the canal with a material that is inert and easy to handle. The most widespread and scientifically accepted root canal filling material is gutta percha, the coagulated sap of certain tropical trees. (See Chapter 11.)

In the early 1950s a Swiss dentist, Dr. Angelo Sargenti, developed a root canal filling material he called N2. The active ingredient is paraformaldehyde, which, in contact with moisture, forms formaldehyde, a potent tissue toxin used in embalming fluid. Paraformaldehyde pastes have not been proved safe, and their use has led to a number of serious complications.

N2 is easier and faster to use than conventional gutta percha, but the pressure needed to get the paste to the very tip of the root can force the mixture into the jawbone beyond the tooth. Recently, a Florida woman received a $1 million judgment from a dentist who had used the Sargenti technique. The N2 injured the left side of her lower jaw, requiring more than forty corrective surgeries.

Another disadvantage of the N2 technique is that when it sets is gets very hard and may be impossible to remove. If some infection still remains in the canal and the root canal has to be redone, the hardened N2 may make the situation uncorrectable. It also makes it more difficult to prepare and place a post restoration.

Despite these considerations, more than thirty thousand dentists in the United States and Canada use N2 or a similar paste-filler, according to the Sargenti-promoting group called the American Endodontic Society. The society provides their members with an impressive plaque, but this wall decoration is misleading and, one might say, unethical, since the officially recognized specialty-certifying group is the American Association of Endodontists.

In 1993 a government advisory panel rejected clinical data that had been submitted to the FDA to demonstrate the claimed safety and effectiveness of N2. The panel found the data flawed and insufficient to support the claims.

SYMPTOMS ALLEGEDLY CAUSED
BY ROOT CANAL THERAPY

We recently received a patient newsletter called "Alternatives." The lead article, based on *Root Canal Cover-Up Exposed,* a book by a dentist, claimed that all teeth that have received root canal therapy are dangerous due to unresolved and constant infections around the root tips. These infections are alleged to cause widespread symptoms.

The theories that this book is based on are without a shred of scientific support and the fanatical recommendation that all teeth with root canal therapy should be extracted is without *any* scientific support. These recommendations, if taken seriously, lead to a particularly vicious form of quackery, the mutilation and crippling of healthy mouths for profit. We have no appropriate words for this brutal and heartless quackery.

ODDBALL TREATMENTS

Some of the oddball treatments listed below are so scientifically ludicrous, and so far removed from the scope of dental practice, that it is hard to believe that any dentist would consider them as serious treatment options. Yet they have been taught to dentists on the postgraduate level and are being used for profit in some dental offices. This brings up a serious legal question, since medical claims are being made that seem clearly beyond the boundaries or competence of traditional dental practice. These dental quacks are practicing medicine without a license.

"Eastern Medicine" and Acupuncture

Acupuncture is based on the ancient Chinese philosophical and mystical viewpoint of life. The body's vital energy—called *chi*—is claimed to circulate through channels in the body called meridians. Interruption of the flow of *chi* leads to illness and disease. "Balance," and therefore health, can be restored by sticking needles in the body at acupuncture points along the meridians to facilitate the flow of *chi*. Originally there were 365 acupoints, a constancy between the human body and the calendar year, but eventually more than 2,000 acupoints were described. Meridians and acupoints have never been anatomically demonstrated or identified.

The acupuncture fad in this country began when *New York Times* reporter James Reston had surgery for appendicitis while visiting China. It was reported that Reston had acupuncture during his treatment, and it was widely assumed that acupuncture was used as an anesthetic during his operation. However, a close reading of his report shows that the acupuncture was not used during the operation but only the day after surgery. The next day Reston was beset with gas pains, common after appendectomies, and inquired about acupuncture. By way of demonstration they stuck him with acupuncture needles, and his gas pains got better, which would have happened whether he had used acupuncture, fondled voodoo dolls, or done nothing.

Evidence for the effectiveness of acupuncture is equivocal. Dr. William Jarvis, of the National Council Against Health Fraud, has pointed out that the best results for acupuncture come from the sloppiest studies, while the careful double-blind studies show no results. In 1990 a Dutch review of acupuncture research concluded that "the quality of even the better studies proved to be mediocre. . . . The efficacy of acupuncture in the treatment of chronic pain remains doubtful."

Apologists for "Eastern medicine" argue that "you can't test Eastern medicine with Western methods." We are supposed to believe that human physiology and the laws of nature change once we cross the international date line. The following is an example of the lengths to which acupuncture apologists will go to give scientific credence to their position. It has been proposed that acupuncture stimulates the formation of pain-relieving chemicals called endorphins. An experiment was designed to demonstrate this, and a noted skeptic was invited to observe. A rabbit was hooked up to an apparatus that measured endorphin levels. The experimenters placed an acupuncture needle in the rabbit, and the gauge on the apparatus duly indicated a small endorphin increase. Another needle was placed, and the needle on the apparatus again moved slightly. At this point the skeptic leaned over and firmly pinched the rabbit, and the gauge needle shot to the end of the scale! The skeptic duly reported that the experiment showed that acupuncture was almost as effective as a pinch on the behind.

Of course, anyone with a background in biology should know that any irritant, be it a needle or a pinch on the behind, will raise the endorphin blood level.

Today we have instruments sensitive enough to detect transmissions from deep outer space, but our instruments have not been able to detect acupuncture meridians, acupoints, or *chi*. The ancients had very incomplete knowledge of anatomy, physiology, or pharmacology. *Chi,* and meridians, were *guesses* about how the body worked. We'll bet if the ancient wise men were somehow transferred to today's world and given access to modern information, they would toss away their ancient theories in a trice.

Auriculotherapy is acupuncture of the ear and is based on the notion that the entire body and internal organs are mapped on the surface of the ear. Proponents claim that it's effective against facial pain and ailments throughout the body. Practitioners insert and twirl needles or, sometimes, just administer small electrical shocks to points on the ear which, they claim, represent the diseased organ. Courses on auriculotherapy are popular among holistic dentists. Although complications from unsterilized and broken needles have been reported, this bizarre method is touted in dental brochures as "quick, easy, inexpensive, effective and completely reversible." A controlled study of auriculotherapy found it to be no more effective against chronic pain than placebo stimulation (light touching).

Always remember that dentists are not trained or licensed to diagnose or treat systemic medical problems.

Applied Kinesiology

Promoters of the theory of applied kinesiology claim that every organ dysfunction is accompanied by a specific muscle weakness, which enables diseases to be diagnosed by testing the strength of a patient's muscles rather than by conventional diagnostic techniques. These promoters—most of them chiropractors or TMJ quacks—also claim that nutritional deficiencies, allergies, and other adverse reactions to food substances can be detected by placing small amounts of the foods in the patient's mouth and then testing for muscle strength. "Good" substances make specific muscles stronger, while "bad" substances lead to muscle weakness. Altering the bite also produces greater muscle strength. Dentists who share these beliefs typically test muscle strength by having their patients hold an arm parallel to the floor. The dentist pushes down on the extended arm to determine its strength. Then, after placing vitamins under the patient's tongue or a piece of plastic between his teeth, again the dentist pushes down on the arm, invariably finding that the arm is "stronger" and that the body will benefit from the vitamins or the plastic mouthpiece. "Treatment" consists of selling expensive vitamin supplements or a plastic appliance. These appliances cost perhaps $20 to make; some dentists charge many hundreds of dollars, or even much more, for these generally useless devices.

Several investigators have tested the theory of applied kinesiology with controlled experiments. One investigator found no difference in muscle response from one substance to another, while another found no difference between the results with test substances and with placebos. The quack value of this procedure is that the results are entirely controllable by the dentist, so patients can be told they're sick or better, depending on how much money the dentist thinks he can squeeze from the patient. Believe it or not, many patients accept expensive, unnecessary, and possibly dangerous treatments based on this silly and disproven diagnostic technique.

Several years ago we attended a course on TMJ given by a famous promoter of applied kinesiology. This lecturer described how he could tell if a crown would fit not by placing it in the patient's mouth, but rather by placing it in one of the patient's hands and then pushing down on the other arm until the arm felt "strong." When some of the dentists in the room started to giggle, ourselves included, we were yelled at by the majority of attendees for being "closed minded." But, as Carl Sagan has pointed out, there is a difference between an open mind and a gaping mind.

Cranial Osteopathy (CO)

The skull is made up of several bones which, beginning in the fetus and ending in childhood, become tightly and immovably attached to one another, so that the skull appears to be one solid block of bone. Despite this, dentists who practice CO claim that these skull bones not only move but that by manipulating them the "energy of life" flows and all kinds of diseases and problems can be cured or prevented. The most sensitive scientific instruments, which can measure movements of a fraction of a micron, have been unable to detect any movement of these skull bones. But we are supposed to believe that the sensitive fingers of those who practice CO not only can easily detect these "movements" but can also treat them. The "treatment" is accomplished by forcibly pushing on the skull. This therapy not only is a waste of the patient's money but also can cause bruising of the head and face.

Reflexology

Reflexology is the diagnosis and treatment of disease by dentists who examine and massage the soles of the feet. Incredible as it sounds, this actually is being promoted at dental meetings. Reflexology is also known as "zone therapy," because advocates claim: (1) the body is divided into ten zones that begin or end in the hands and feet; (2) each organ or part of the body is represented on the hands and feet; (3) the practitioner can diagnose abnormalities by feeling the feet; and (4) massaging or pressing an area can stimulate the flow of energy, blood, nutrients, and nerve impulses to the corresponding body zone. There is no scientific evidence to support these claims. Reflexology is also promoted as being successful in reducing stress. Because foot massage can be relaxing, this claim probably has validity. However, there is no reason to pay high fees to a dentist to provide this service.

Halitosis

Some dentists have found bad breath to be very profitable. An ad in a dental practice management magazine states: "You can cash in on one of the hottest opportunities right now in dentistry . . . The diagnosis and treatment of breath disorders . . . Increase your net income by $10–20,000 per month!" Halitosis can be caused by a number of things, but the dentists who have set up antihalitosis centers as part of their practices or, in a few cases, separate clinics "specializing" in bad breath, have no special knowledge concerning the diagnosis or treatment of this condition. They are, in fact, concerned mostly with increasing their profit margins by selling scientifically unproven products. At this time there is no single product that can be used to "cure" all kinds of breath odor problems. (See Chapter 17.)

Lasers and Headaches

Some dentists claim they can successfully treat migraine headaches with low-power lasers. There is no evidence to support this. (See Chapter 17.)

Cavitational Osteopathosis and Biological Dentistry

Some dentists claim that facial pain and even pains throughout the body are caused by infected "cavities" within the jawbones. These cavities are not detectable on X-ray examination and are not treatable with antibiotics. They are not abscesses, cysts, or lesions, all of which are detectable with X rays. Certain dentists believe that they can somehow find these cavities and, by surgically scraping them out, cure the infection and resolve the pain. This alleged condition is called cavitational osteopathosis; there is no scientific evidence to support this assertion or the diagnostic and treatment methods based on it.

Based on the dubious theory behind cavitational osteopathosis, a group of dentists have formed the American Academy of Biological Dentistry. Postgraduate seminars given, for profit, by this organization have persuaded a number of dentists and some physicians to claim that they can cure diseases such as arthritis, heart disease, and pain throughout the body by finding and removing infected cavities within the patient's jawbones.

Believers in biological dentistry have taken the treatment one step farther—they also remove all root-canal-treated teeth and most of the vital teeth close to the area where they say an infection exists. According to a 1994 article in *Milwaukee Magazine,* a group of local patients filed suit against several practitioners of this bizarre and dangerous therapy. These patients had numerous perfectly healthy teeth removed without any improvement in their diseases, and the state licensing board is also investigating. Unfortunately, this is not the end of the story. The biological dentistry movement is still strong, and we often receive brochures touting meetings and continuing education courses. If your dentist tells you that a systemic disease or pains far from the mouth are due to infected jawbone cavities, run fast and find another dentist!

Craniosacral Therapy

About twenty years ago a fringe group of osteopaths developed a treatment called craniosacral therapy base on a bizarre theory of how the body works. They proposed that a rhythm exists for the flow of the fluid that surrounds our brain and spinal cord and that they could diagnose disease by feeling for aberrations in this rhythm and correct the aberrations by proper manipulation. Today a number of dentists and physical therapists have adopted this theory.

A course brochure for craniosacral therapy for dentists states: "CranioSacral Therapy is used to treat a myriad of health problems, including headaches, neck and back pain, TMJ dysfunction, chronic fatigue, motor coordination difficulties, eye problems, endogenous depression, hyperactivity, and central nervous system disorders. It is a gentle, non-invasive, hands-on technique that, helps detect and correct an imbalance in the CranioSacral System, which may be the cause of sensory, motor, or intellectual dysfunction."

A 1994 well-controlled study of this theory failed to support it. In a commentary following the article a distinguished professor of physical therapy stated: "Basically, clinicians should not try to measure something unless they know what that something is." This is good advice and would well be heeded by those making some of the silly claims involved with diagnosing and treating chronic pain.

Homeopathy

At first glance, homeopathy is so silly that it appears to be a joke. The aphorist Ambrose Bierce, at the beginning of the century, defined a *homeopath* as "the humorist of the medical profession."

Homeopathy was invented by a German physician, Samuel Hahneman, in the late 1700s. Hahneman was justifiably distressed about the leechings, purgings, bloodlettings, poisonings (due to toxic medications), and other invasive medical procedures of his day. Medicine at that time was termed "heroic," possibly because you had to be a hero to undergo treatment. Hahneman believed that common medical practice did more harm than good, and he developed a noninvasive system of medicine, called homeopathy, which avoided the havoc that heroic medicine produced but also was scientifically unsound. In disrepute for years, homeopathy is making a comeback.

Homeopathy states that the more dilute a medication is, the more powerful it becomes. Advocates of homeopathy believe that if you go to the beach and throw an aspirin in the ocean you can come back a year later, take a sip, and cure your headache. This is not an exaggeration; the dilutions in homeopathic remedies really are of this order. Of course, this homeopathic theory is the exact opposite of what pharmacologists have demonstrated time and time again with every known medication: For every drug there is a clearly defined dose-response relationship in which increasing the dose increases the effect. Belief in homeopathy requires that we throw out all current knowledge of chemistry and pharmocology.

The 1938 Federal Food, Drug, and Cosmetic Act gave homeopathic remedies legal acceptance without requiring prior scrutiny by the FDA. This statute was shepherded through Congress by Senator Royal Copeland (D-NY), a prominent homeopathic physician, and is still on the books. In 1990 a review of homeopathic research concluded that there was no evidence that homeopathy had any more value than placebo therapy.

Chiropractic

Many chiropractors are treating patients with TMD, often in collaboration with a dentist. As one chiropractic brochure says: "Because the problem of TMJ dysfunction often involves both spinal and dental components, the most satisfying results for you will be found using a comprehensive interdisciplinary approach of dentistry and chiropractic."

The basic theory of chiropractic, that nerve interference is a major cause of disease, has been consistently rejected by the scientific community because it does not conform to established anatomical facts and has not been supported by properly done controlled studies. We believe that chiropractors should not be treating facial pain patients; the potential for misdiagnosis and improper treatment is great.

Faith Healing

There is a faith healer who claims to change silver fillings into gold. Of course he is a fraud. Faith healing is perhaps the cruelest quackery of them all. A sick patient, after scraping up a contribution to the wealthy faith healer, finds after a few days that he is still just as sick. He now realizes that no matter how devout he is, and how much he loves God, God spurns him, because he is not cured as was promised by the faith healer. Now not only does he still have his disease to contend with, but he must live with the knowledge that God despises him. The ordinary quack takes your money and your health and perhaps your life. The faith healer takes all the above and the most precious consolation of them all, the faith and comfort of God's love.

PLACEBOS

Skeptics always claim that an unexpected medical success from an avant-garde therapy, Lourdes to laetrile, is due to the placebo effect, but very few people understand what a placebo really is.

We usually think of placebos as sugar pills, things that confuse the minds of those less intelligent than we are but that could never fool us. But that's not accurate. A nonspecific effect (placebo) is a response resulting from the *act of treatment* rather than from the treatment itself. Research into the psychological consequences of what are now called nonspecific effects proves that placebos are much more involved in healing than we once thought. It's not that some simple people are easily fooled. All of us exhibit some level of nonspecific effects every time we undergo any kind of treatment, even when the only treatment is the assurance that we'll get better.

Recovery from illness, whether it follows self-medication, legitimate treatment, or bogus therapies, may lead one to conclude that the treatment received was the cause of the return of good health. By now you recognize this as a logical fallacy, a conclusion that does not follow from the premise. The "return of good health" may be a result of the placebo effect.

In 1955, the groundbreaking "The Powerful Placebo" was published. This paper is probably responsible for the double-blind study design being universally adopted as the gold standard for research. The paper reported that the average placebo response rate was 35.2 percent, and it's this figure that leads to the common statement that one-third of the population responds to placebos. But recent research has shown that the figure is considerably higher.

Even effective treatments can be influenced by the doctor's or patient's attitude toward the therapy, and no treatment, from antibiotics to surgery, is without some level of nonspecific effect. Separating valid therapies from invalid ones is obviously difficult. This explains why testimonials and anecdotes are scientifically worthless substitutes for controlled experiments. The fact that your cold symptoms improved after a bowl of your grandmother's chicken soup reflects your grandmother's love and tender care, not any secret or magical ingredient in her soup. And a cold gets better anyway. Anytime you hear or see an ad featuring someone giving a testimonial touting some therapy, think of the placebo effect and be wary!

Later research confirmed the earlier findings and established that the more complicated the placebo, the greater the placebo effect. Patients told to take ordinary-looking placebo pills on a routine schedule showed the common placebo effect, but patients given different-colored pills, and instructed to take them on a complicated schedule, did significantly better.

There are also a number of other myths associated with placebos. Try to answer these questions:

- Does a positive response to a placebo mean that your problem is imaginary?
- Do you have to believe in treatment for a placebo effect to occur?
- Are placebos harmless?

The answer to all three questions is no. Placebo responses can appear in patients with true illnesses. The subjective symptoms (such as pain) can resolve, making the patient feel better, while the objective symptoms (such as low blood count, fever, muscle weakness) remain. And while a patient may not believe a treatment can help, on another, perhaps subconscious, level he may hopefully welcome the treatment. Although most people believe placebos are safe, they can be dangerous. A quack, relying on the placebo response, can string along a genuinely sick person and dangerously delay urgently needed appropriate treatment.

Quack dentists are usually well aware of the placebo effect, and they use it to deceive and cheat unwary patients. The dentist who removes silver fillings to treat systemic disease is depending on the placebo effect to make the patient feel better and credit the improvement to a wonderful and compassionate dentist. Holistic dentists in particular are unwilling to accept the placebo effect as an explanation for any of their successes; rather they invent all kinds of energies, auras, and scenarios to fit in with their phony but profitable treatment strategies.

The use of placebos is not innocent. Doctors who employ (and usually sell) placebo therapies to treat such nonexistant diseases as "reactive hypoglycemia," phony yeast infections, or amalgam "toxicity" often become gurus to their patients, who in turn are generally taught that their particular "disease" can be treated only by a specific therapy employed by their own special and unique practitioner. On the other hand, the promoter of a placebo can be blinded to the presence of real and life-threatening illness, because of the belief that the patient's symptoms are only imagined. In addition, placebos have been known to trigger allergic-type reactions such as a massive swelling of the face, particularly the lips.

The question has been raised that, since the placebo effect is so pronounced, why doesn't the legitimate doctor make use of it? The answer is that legitimate doctors do indeed utilize the placebo effect, but in a sound medical context. As eminent pain researcher Dr. Joseph Marbach has pointed out, the doctor should know if he is using a placebo. The very worst scenario is when both the patient and the doctor are unaware that a placebo is being used. (This is not what we mean when we talk of a "double-blind study.")

This information should convince you how difficult it is to separate fact from fiction when investigating different medical therapies. We recommend that you continue to enjoy your grandmother's chicken soup but that you realize that some of the good results from the soup or any other kind of treatment are due to those pesky, confusing, and ubiquitous placebos.

THE PROMOTION AND PROPAGATION
OF DENTAL QUACKERY

Dentistry is still, basically, a cottage industry with the vast majority of dentists working in private and solo practice. This allows dentists to perform unproven therapies without criticism from knowledgeable colleagues. Many dental quacks truly believe in the techniques they're promoting. The instruction of dental students is at fault. The ADA's former director of scientific affairs, commenting about dental education, has said, "The very things that would explicate the scientific method—animal experimentation, for example—have been deleted for the most part. Also, virtually no dental student is compelled to read a sampling of good scientific articles, which would help clarify how science progresses from one point to the next."

On the postgraduate level, quality control in the selection of courses and lecturers is often nonexistent. And although most postgraduate and continuing education courses are valid, unproven and disproven topics are far more common than they should be. Boston University's Goldman School of Dentistry has sponsored continuing education courses for dentists that feature such marvels of modern science as reflexology, acupressure, and auriculotherapy. Georgetown Dental School has offered an expensive postgraduate course in cranial osteopathy. The Greater New York Dental Meeting has sponsored quack courses, and many local state dental journals have published articles on unscientific and disproven treatments.

The 1995 Greater Long Island Dental Meeting included a course on Chinese medicine, approved for continuing education credit and taught by a chiropractor, that recommended various oddball treatments and suggested that intuition (of all things) be used to make a diagnosis. The instructor was disparaging about medicines but enthusiastic about the use of herbs, possibly not realizing that herbs are also medicines (and ones that are not standardized or tested). We are always eager to learn new procedures and better ways to practice dentistry. But we insist that they be based on science.

Some of these and similar courses have received accreditation by the ADA and the Academy of General Dentistry. When a prestigious school or dental group gives a course good for postgraduate credit it is easy to conclude mistakenly that the material of the course is scientifically valid. We have long petitioned the ADA to set standards for continuing education courses. Such complaints to the American Dental Association have resulted in the formation of the Continuing Education Recognition Program, but we have found CERP to be worthless in screening out courses of poor quality. (See Chapter 2.) CERP seems to be a rubber-stamp committee, and it has approved sponsors of courses promoting unscientific and disproven subjects such as homeopathy. Of course the ADA is also concerned that aggressive action by them could trigger expensive lawsuits. And, finally, since lectures are profitable, many sponsors are unwilling to restrict them at all.

Several years ago a group of dentists who promote the use of scientifically unproven TMJ diagnostic and treatment devices sued the ADA to prohibit a scientific meeting sponsored by the ADA that would have attempted to establish guidelines for TMJ therapy. Concerned that their pet gadgets would not withstand close scientific scrutiny, they used the threat of a lawsuit to prevent the ADA from publishing any conclusions unfavorable to their devices. These conclusions would have helped protect the public from many unproven and dangerous treatments and quack devices. The case never went to court, because the typically timid ADA capitulated before the threats.

Much is being made of the National Institutes of Health awarding some small grants to study some of these "alternative" treatments. The holistic fringe is triumphantly trumpeting this as if it legitimized their claims. Generally speaking, reputable scientists do not waste their time examining claims that run counter to established scientific principles; we know of no geologists who are trying to prove that Earth is flat. But there has been considerable political pressure put on the NIH by the quack establishment and by certain congresspeople who may be scientifically illiterate but have a keen nose for campaign contributions. We assume the NIH expects that, once an investigation disproves a quack claim, the clamor will go away. We doubt it. Quackery is too easy and too lucrative to go away quietly.

THE MEDIA AND QUACKERY

The media have played a particularly malignant role in the propagation of quackery. There are many examples of the media actually promoting fraudulent medical schemes to the public. The notorious 1990 *60 Minutes* program that promoted the discredited claims of antiamalgam "researchers" sent thousands of Americans to be mutilated at the hands of anti-amalgam quacks. Another regrettable TV segment featured a man who claimed he had been infected with AIDS at his dentist's office. His evidence was that he couldn't imagine where else he could have contracted the disease! This same program showed an experiment with dental equipment that was a joke to anyone familiar with dental instruments and the requirements of a scientific experiment.

Then there is the case of a famous football quarterback who was injured before an important playoff game. His doctors forbade him to play, but the newspapers headlined that he would indeed play because he was treated successfully by electro-acupuncture. He did play in the game, very briefly, and he never played again. The media gave favorable publicity to electro-acupuncture but never reported that this "alternative" treatment encouraged him to play against his doctor's orders, resulting in injury that ended his career.

As a direct consequence of the *60 Minutes* program, monies were allocated for a Public Health Service study of silver-amalgam fillings. The study was published in 1993 and concluded that "there are no data to compel a change in the current use of dental amalgam." This echoes the conclusions of every responsible study done on the subject. *60 Minutes* never aired a retraction of the false anti-amalgam story, and this segment is still used by quacks to convince patients to have their perfectly good silver fillings removed.

It would be most desirable from every standpoint if the American Dental Association would take the lead in battling dental quackery. But the ADA has recently abandoned all pretenses of trying to regulate the behavior of its members or of the manufacturers of quack dental devices and materials. The ADA has adopted this sorry posture partly because of a fear of lawsuits. Should the ADA officially criticize a treatment or a device, it will cost the proponents and purveyors of such methods business, and they will sue the ADA. In this country it seems to be illegal to interfere with anyone's profits, even if he is selling phony goods and services. So, for the moment, or until the ADA develops some backbone and is willing to stand up to the quacks, the public cannot count on the organization of the American dental profession for protection against dental quacks.

The best defense against quackery is an understanding of how scientific knowledge is developed and verified. Your dentist should be willing to explain treatment options and whether any suggested treatment goes contrary to accepted norms, and why. You must judge if the dentist's explanations are consistent with scientific method. You can and should seek second and third opinions when extensive dentistry is being proposed.

If the dentist promises to treat medical conditions, or claims special knowledge or skills not held by colleagues, or claims to prevent future medical problems, or uses any methods not in general use, you are best advised to beware!

IF YOU ARE A VICTIM

If you believe you've been a victim of dental quackery, you may be able to do something about it. Contact your local dental society, the office of professional conduct, and the attorney general; these should be listed in your telephone directory. You can also contact the Victim Redress Committee of the National Council Against Health Fraud, c/o Michael Botts, Esq., P.O. Box 187, Prescott, WI 54021.

Part IV

*

Insurance and Managed Care

21. Third-Party Reimbursement

*

So much of what we call management consists in making it difficult for people to work.
— PETER DRUCKER

T he health care system in America is proving to be a muddle of inequities, bureaucracy, paperwork, fraud, and incompetence. Honest and competent health care providers, drowning in paperwork and contradictory bureaucratic regulations, are finding it difficult to do their jobs satisfactorily. Most proposals for reform are opposed by self-interest groups for various reasons, but a consensus seems to be forming that it is more than time for reform, even if it means a radical overhaul of the traditional health care delivery system. And proposals for reform, no matter how much they differ, are being lumped under the euphemistic but politically euphonious name "managed care." All managed care proposals, however they differ, share the same premise: Reducing the amount of compensation will force "providers" (physicians, dentists, etc.) to eliminate waste and become more efficient, thus lowering costs and making decent care available to all. Politically this is irresistible, but unfortunately, the principles behind managed care do not work. This is not to say that reform is impossible; reform is not only necessary but also very possible. It has been said that simply eliminating quackery and fraud from the professions will save so many *billions* that the problems would be solved then and there.

We believe that dentistry is the logical profession to lead the way to reform. The goals and methods of dentistry are more straightforward than are those of medicine and more susceptible to analysis and subsequent reform. Reforms in the incentives and delivery systems of dentistry could then be modified to fit the more complex problems of the medical delivery system as a whole.

For generations details of treatment and conditions of payment were strictly the business of the dentist and the patient. This has changed dramatically in the last decades with the intrusion of third parties into the doctor-patient relationship. The doctor and the patient are the first two parties; the third party is someone else, perhaps a union, an insurance company, a government agency, or an employer. In these new plans the third party provides financing, sometimes facilities, and often even the doctor. These plans can be bought as private insurance policies, but much more often they are provided by the private sector or government as fringe benefits in employment contracts. Politically, they are given as part of the welfare or social security systems, either to assist those who cannot afford to pay for treatment (Medicaid) or as general entitlements to older citizens (Medicare). At this writing Medicare does not include dental care, but the indigent nationwide are covered for some dental work by Medicaid. For the rest of the country, private third-party dental plans have become very popular: Well over 100 million people in the United States, over 40 percent of the population, have some private dental insurance. These plans are socially and politically attractive, seemingly bringing us closer to the ideal of universal health care. But as these plans proliferate, many serious mistakes have been made.

ERRORS IN PLANNING

One of the mistakes third parties have made is the application of traditional insurance techniques to dentistry. The insurance industry calculates costs by averaging per-person expenditures and multiplying by the number of people expected to be covered. This works in medicine, but not in dentistry, because in dentistry per-capita expenditure does not reflect per-capita *need*. In medicine, need is usually transient, but dental need is often chronic and enduring. For too many Americans this need is overwhelming: The mouth is in such poor shape that the patient is overwhelmed by the contemplated expense and inconvenience of needed treatment and will wait until the mouth completely falls apart and dentures are needed. Many won't even get dentures, and, with a couple of snaggly teeth, will survive on soft food. Dental need is not life-threatening, and very often needed treatment is deferred because of finances, apathy, or fear. In the population there is a huge backlog of dental need, unlike in medicine, where a sick person usually sees a doctor, recovers by himself, or dies. In dentistry unattended need remains for years; a missing tooth unreplaced will be missing years later. A person newly covered by medical insurance does not run out to have his appendix removed or have brain surgery. But the person newly covered by dental insurance is likely to have that $20,000 rehabilitation done.

Need is one thing; *demand* is something else. Insurance premiums traditionally are calculated from *demand* as measured by expenditure. In medicine, need is related to disability and discomfort and is often perceived as life-threatening, so demand closely approaches need. But in dentistry demand and need are far apart; need is not life-threatening or disabling. So at first insurers were losing money on dental coverage. A premium set at a few hundred dollars did not cover costs if subscribers were already carrying around a backlog of dental need that would cost thousands to correct. So these plans have been drastically amended. Premiums have been raised sharply and benefits reduced, and co-payments (the patient paying part of the doctor's fee) have been instituted and increased. Prior approval requirements were started. Some third parties went over to "closed-end" plans that did not allow the patient to use his own dentist: coverage was provided only if the patient used one of a panel of dentists who had agreed to accept low fees. (The insurer felt that cheaper dentists would cost the insurer less. But, as we shall see, it doesn't work that way.)

Where prior approval is required, the dentist has to send a description of planned extensive treatment along with the patient's X rays to the insurer. The insurer's dental consultants screen planned treatments and eliminate those deemed unnecessary or excessive, or those not covered by the contract. But short-term economies often lead to long-term greater expense. As an example, the insurance consultant following the policy guidelines might select a less-costly treatment that is odds-on to fail in a few years, requiring greater long-range expense.

Here is an illustration of how much more costly in the long run poor dentistry is compared to good dentistry. Suppose a patient has a large cavity in a molar. If the filling is hastily and improperly done, without decay being completely removed, the tooth is likely to abscess, requiring a root canal. If the root canal is improperly done, the tooth is likely to become reinfected and have to be extracted; now a fixed bridge is needed. If that is hastily done, with poor marginal fit, poor bite, and the other sins of badly done bridgework, the bridge will fail, along with progressive loss of teeth, and be replaced with another bridge, and yet another, and then with a poorly made partial denture, and another, until no teeth are left and a full denture is needed. All of these procedures have to be paid for, and all of these costs would have been unnecessary had the right job been done at the right time. At any point along this chain, good dentistry could have put an end to this dismal procession of failure. While it is true that a Goodwork filling would have cost somewhat more to begin with, just look at the "bargain" the insurer received from Dr. Poorwork, not to mention the years of pain and inconvenience and the final dental disaster to the patient.

THE POORER THE SERVICE, THE GREATER THE REWARD

The fee schedules for the various third-party plans provide powerful economic incentives to do the wrong thing. As an example, fees allowed for fillings are typically very low, while fees allowed for extractions are much higher. A dentist confronted with a tooth requiring a complicated and difficult filling may well be tempted to tell the patient that the tooth can't be saved, especially since the dentist will earn more for the couple of minutes it takes to do the extraction than for the better part of an hour he would have to spend to do the filling properly. And once the tooth is out, probably along with other teeth sharing the same fate, the dentist might opt to make a partial denture, which, according to the insurance plan, is more lucrative, easier, and requires less time than do other and better treatment options.

Probably the most shortsighted money-saving scheme is the closed-end-panel plan. Insurers controlling a supply of patients can force dentists who rely on these patients to accept lower fees if they want to remain in the program. This virtually guarantees Poorwork results. Dentists trying to make a profit from the plan's low fees must provide hurry-up, volume, low-quality dentistry and resort to bait and switch and other fraudulent techniques.

There are better answers to problems of high cost than low-fee closed-end panels, but sad to say, these answers are not forthcoming. Instead, many insurers are going to plans that compel the use of closed-end panels. Previously, most dental plans allowed a member the option of seeking good dentistry from his own dentist, with the plan paying part of the dentist's fee and the member paying the rest. But now, many plans do not cover any treatment rendered by a dentist outside of the closed panel. The member has the option of using the closed-panel-plan dentist and seemingly having his treatment completely paid for, or using his old private dentist and, not getting any coverage at all, having to pay the dentist's whole fee. In the latter case the member is faced with having to pay, either directly by salary withholding or through union dues, the premium for coverage he can never use. This is a tremendous incentive for the member to leave his own dentist and use the plan dentist. And, as more patients abandon their long-time dentists for these plans, this becomes a powerful inducement for the long-time dentist to join the plan.

Dr. Fraud's Scams

Plan member patients may be in for a big surprise. The plan dentist may do a few procedures covered by the plan, then suddenly confront the patient with an expensive job that just happens not to be covered. This bait-and-switch technique is common and is almost forced on the plan dentist by economic necessity. In fact, practice management lecturers to dental groups are advising dentists that, before signing up with any plan, they make sure that there are a great many procedures that are not covered by the plan, to give the dentist scope for making a living.

A patient of ours provides a recent example. He had been our patient for three years, then dropped out of sight for the next three years. Recently he called us and asked if we would give him a second opinion. For reasons of economy, he was now going to the closed-panel union dentist. For two years he received perfunctory cleanings, but now the dentist refused to do a cleaning for him, saying he had to see the clinic periodontist. The periodontist told him he needed full-mouth periodontal surgery, at a cost of $4,000, and, as it happened, the surgery was not included in the plan. When we examined his mouth we found that the patient's lower jaw was in excellent periodontal condition, needing just an ordinary cleaning, while the upper jaw had two teeth that required deep scaling. No surgery was needed at all. Here is a case where the closed-end clinic used not only bait and switch but also outright fraud. That this was typical of many other instances that have come to our attention is not surprising, since the low fees forced upon these dentists almost make it necessary to commit fraud in order to survive economically.

In a more recent example, another patient of ours decided she would use the union clinic, since she "was paying for it anyway." She had some pain in a tooth but had to wait a few weeks to get an appointment at the union clinic. She was examined, two X rays were taken, and she was told that her pain was caused by gum disease, and she would need surgery and other expensive treatments that were not covered (sound familiar?). She came to us for another opinion. By this time her pain had become severe, and an X ray showed that the pain was caused by an obvious, easily diagnosed deep cavity in the offending tooth. Had this cavity been treated promptly and properly, when the symptoms first started, it was probable that a relatively simple filling would have solved the problem. But now, after the refusal of the clinic to treat the cavity and the subsequent delay, her tooth had become infected (abscessed) and would need root canal treatment and a post and crown restoration, all major and expensive dentistry. When we told the patient what had happened, she screamed, "How do they get away with that? That's criminal!"

We agree. But who are the criminals? Surely the dentists in the clinics are to blame, but we feel strongly that this guilt must be shared by the union officials who contracted with this clinic to pay their dentists such low fees that they are virtually forced to defraud in order to make a living. And what about the role played by the social engineers and their well-meaning but empty-headed managed care plans?

And how do we feel about the young dentist, up to his ears in debt from his schooling, who finds out that in order to find a job, in order to practice the profession he has learned and invested so heavily in, he must accept a situation where, to squeeze out an adequate income, he must conspire to defraud his patients?

THE YOUNG DENTIST AND MANAGED CARE

We have interviewed dentists who have been employed in these clinics. Conditions do vary, but some generalizations apply to many of them.

The dentists are paid on commission. Since the designated-plan fees are small to begin with, commissions on these small fees are even smaller, giving a powerful incentive to the dentist to speed up his work or even fraudulently report more work than was done. There are no checks on either quality or fraud, and therefore no restraints on these practices. One dentist reported that if he scaled half the patient's mouth and reported it honestly, the clinic owner would fraudulently report that the other half was also done. Ironically, the dentist's commission would be only on the half mouth scaled; the owner would pocket the entire fee for the falsely reported other half.

Patients were looked on as an opportunity to make money, not as an opportunity to provide a needed service to a human being. When a patient was in the dental chair for treatment, the clinic dentist would do everything possible for that patient in one sitting, largely because the patient might not come back for the next visit, and a moneymaking opportunity would be lost. If the insurance plan would allow, the patient might get four quadrants of scaling, many fillings, several root canals from start to finish, and even some posts screwed in and teeth prepared for crowns. One can imagine the ghastly quality of service resulting from such haste!

One dentist at a clinic routinely reported, for each patient he treated, doing four-surface fillings on every back tooth in the mouth, whether or not they were needed and whether or not they were actually done.

The clinic had a book detailing the specifics of coverage for every insurance program. Some insurance plans actively invited fraud. One plan allowed for complete deep scaling and periodontal root planing, fluoride treatments, and polishing on the same visit. The dentists might just take a rotary brush and briefly polish the teeth, then claim all the above procedures. The patient charts were color-coded to differentiate from Medicaid, insurance plans, and the occasional private cash patient. Surprisingly, the cash patients were not considered desirable because fraudulent reporting was not possible; the cash patient would complain if charged for things that were not done. Insurance and Medicaid patients gave more scope for profit.

FEE FOR SERVICE

The classic comment about fee-for-service health care was made by George Bernard Shaw, who asked, "How would you like to be brought up on charges before a judge who wouldn't be paid unless he found you guilty?"

Fee-for-service programs can be sponsored by employers or unions, or purchased by groups or individuals. Fee-for-service means that the provider of the service gets paid a specific fee for a specific service. Treating a throat, filling a tooth, and trimming a toenail are all services for which specific fees are set. This has been the historic basis for computing health care fees.

The intrusion of third parties into the health care picture has led to complications that strongly magnify the shortcomings of fee-for-service. At first, third-party plans were generally based on fee-for-service because it has been the traditional method of compensation and because it seems to reward diligence and industry on the part of the providers (the doctors who provide the services). But how it has worked in practice is something else, since diligence and industry translate to the actuarial term "production," and when the provider is being paid for a number representing "production," the incentive is to maximize, one way or another, that number. This can lead to the overemphasis of not-needed but reimbursable procedures and the neglect of necessary but unrewarded treatments. A major factor is the incentive to speed up work so as to report more "production" and receive more compensation. Of course, speed is the death of quality. This failing of fee-for-service can be corrected only by a serious and effective system of quality assurance.

Originally these programs were quite comprehensive, with most dental procedures covered and with fees considered adequate by many dentists. But quality assurance was not built into these programs, and too many dentists abused the programs with over-utilization, poor quality, and/or outright fraud. The response by the insurance industry was to increase subscriber cost, decrease the dollar amount of coverage per specified service, and increase the number of services not covered. A preferred industry response would have been to try to eliminate incompetence, over-utilization, fraud, and quackery.

In an attempt to control costs, many policies request, and some require, pretreatment forms to be submitted, ostensibly to inform patients whether planned treatment will be covered but possibly simply to add another delaying tactic and more paperwork. Perhaps it would be more sensible to require occasional post-treatment checkups with impartial experts to see if treatment was properly done. This way the carrier could decline to pay for substandard treatment that offers poor prognosis. At the present time many insurance carriers will pay to replace a filling every three years and a crown every five years. This reflects experience with the substandard dentistry that the design of the policies invites. Good-quality dentistry shows sharply differing results: Studies of silver filling longevity have shown a thirteen-year survival rate of 90 percent. We often see fillings that are twenty-five to fifty years old and even older. Well-made crowns show equally great longevity. It should be obvious that it is more cost-effective to pay somewhat more for a restoration that might last a lifetime than to pay less for a job that has to be redone every three years. It is silly for a program to pay for the poor prognosis offered by poor treatment, when it can insist on the good prognosis promised by high quality, even if the high-quality treatment is more expensive at the outset.

Pretreatment requirements often lead to other problems. A dentist planning to do a complex but necessary restoration may find out that the insurance examiner rejects coverage for this treatment and suggests an "alternative" treatment. Invariably the suggested alternative is inferior and will not serve the patient nearly as well as the dentist's plan, but it is a whole lot cheaper. Once we called a plan's examining dentist to complain that his suggestion would lead to inevitable loss of the patient's remaining teeth, while our plan would retain healthy function much longer. "If the patient were your wife or your daughter," we asked this dentist, "would you do what we suggested or what you did?"

"I would use your treatment, of course," was his prompt answer. "But we don't provide Cadillacs to everyone." This kind of thinking is understandable, if the alternative were a reasonable treatment. But in this situation, it wasn't a case of a Cadillac versus a Ford, it was a case of life or death for the patient's teeth. And in this case the patient was being denied the treatment her premiums were supposed to be covering.

These programs often have one set of fees for participating dentists (dentists who have agreed to accept the reimbursement as full payment for covered procedures) and another, lower fee schedule for nonparticipating dentists. This is to encourage dentists to participate in the plan. It can be much more expensive for a patient to go to a nonparticipating dentist than to a participating one. A patient choosing a nonparticipating dentist has to pay the difference in fee between the reimbursement schedule and the dentist's charge. This gives the insurer the opportunity to further manipulate the decision-making process: by pressuring the patient to go to a participating dentist and by pressuring the nonparticipating dentist to cut his fees. The dentist is tempted to pad the insurance forms to restore his own income or to decrease or eliminate the amount of money the patient would have to pay out of pocket. The lower the fee schedule, the more pressure on the dentist to spend less time per procedure, cut corners, and create a profit out of mass-produced, low-quality dentistry. Now many insurers are going to so-called closed-panel plans: If the patient selects a dentist participating in the plan, he receives partial or full coverage, but the patient selecting a nonparticipating dentist receives no coverage at all. We wonder if this is legal. After all, the patient, through union dues or from payroll deductions, is paying premiums for coverage and is being denied the coverage he has paid for if he uses his long-time nonplan dentist. If it's not illegal, it certainly is unfair.

Some of the problems are illustrated by the following examples, all actual cases:

A patient went for a throat exam. The doctor asked a few questions and looked through a nasal probe (a procedure that takes less than a minute). The patient then got a prescription and made a co-payment. A few weeks later the patient got a statement from the third-party carrier (Blue Cross, in this case) that the doctor received nearly $400 for the five-minute visit. The most expensive procedure itemized in the statement was "surgery." When the patient asked the doctor about this, the doctor replied that the scope placed in the nose constituted "surgery."

A patient went to his private dentist who competently and

properly completed a complicated two-surface filling in half an hour. The patient's brother went to another dentist, a member of his union's managed-care plan, who hastily and sloppily performed four similar fillings in half an hour. The third-party carrier paid the second dentist four times as much as it paid the first dentist. The patient of the first dentist complained because he had to pay a small part of his dentist's fee while his brother didn't have to pay anything, and for "four times the number of fillings yet!"

An elderly man went to a podiatrist because he was losing the manual dexterity to cut his toenails, and his friends recommended the podiatrist because "Medicare will pay." The podiatrist spent five minutes trimming the toenails, and Medicare subsequently sent the patient a statement showing that the doctor was paid more than $300 for "surgery." The patient indignantly called the doctor's office to complain and was told, "What do you care? It didn't cost you anything!"

The example of the throat examination is not necessarily health fraud, but it represents the doctor raising his "production" by exploiting an incompetent definition of "surgery" by the carrier. Fee for service tempts the doctor to perform services that generate the most "production," even if these services are unnecessary.

The example of the two dentists illustrates the most glaring and self-defeating defect of fee for service: raising "production" by haste, leading to incompetent performance. The second dentist's work will have to be redone time and again, all at a fee; the treated teeth will ultimately need extractions and replacement, all at larger fees; and the pattern will be repeated until the patient needs dentures and expense has been heavy. All the while the patient of the first dentist has a competent restoration that will last well into the future, expense will be reasonably low, and oral health will be maintained. The dismal spectacle of a third party grossly overpaying for incompetent and harmful treatments while paying the minimum for effective treatment is built into fee-for-service schemes. Again we have that paradox: The poorer the quality of service, the greater the reward to the provider.

The toenail trimming is a simple example of raising "production" by fraud. Fee for service pays for individual services, so the doctor gets paid more if he lists additional services, even if they are not performed. (In this case the patient was indignant but said he was too old to fight City Hall. Many of the podiatrist's elderly patients probably felt the same way. This type of fraud is widespread and rarely caught.) Some insurance experts have estimated that over $100 billion yearly is thrown away on fraudulent overbilling.

Many dentists routinely overcharge by listing procedures as more complex than they actually were. A study by a dental insurance administrator determined that 62 percent of claims for payment by oral surgeons in California contained overcharges. In almost 50 percent of extractions, the surgeons claimed that the procedure used to remove a tooth was more complex and thus more expensive than was justified by the actual surgical procedure that was employed.

CAPITATION

Capitation, which means "by the head," is a reimbursement system in which the doctor gets paid a set sum for each patient enrolled in his list, without regard to how many times, if ever, the patient is seen and regardless of the nature of the treatment provided. This system is used by some countries that have a national health program ("socialized medicine"). The basic idea is that the healthier the patient, the less he requires services, and the more profitable it is for the doctor. Thus, in a dental capitation plan, it is presumed that there is an incentive for the dentist to do the most careful and effective work, so the patient has less trouble and needs to utilize less of the dentist's time and overhead expense.

Unfortunately, this system is even more susceptible to abuse than fee for service. The doctor gets paid the same if he works hard and long with the patient or if he doesn't see the patient at all; the incentive is for the doctor to ignore the patient's complaints and even omit doing important work. The average citizen probably carries around thousands of dollars' worth of untreated dental problems. As mentioned above, these problems are not felt to be urgent or life threatening by the average citizen, and thus they are not treated. However, they are likely to receive attention once insurance will pay the bill.

We know dentists who participate in capitation plans. When confronted with a patient needing expensive restorations, these dentists simply ignore the situation. This is understandable, since the capitation fee given to the dentist doesn't approach what would be the huge costs of comprehensive care. Thus capitation often results in the neglect of the patient's needs. A capitation plan dentist we know was asked what he would do if a patient needed a crown, since the plan paid a fraction of what a crown costs. "I don't do it," was the blunt answer. Indeed, capitation plans make the dentist the patient's insurer, because the dentist is financially responsible for any work the patient requires and will actually lose money if the needed work done is more expensive than the capitated reimbursement.

We believe this is an outright conflict of interest. Whose financial well-being do you think a capitation doctor will select, the patient's or the doctor's? The few studies of dental capitation plans that have been done demonstrate that capitated patients received fewer of the high-overhead procedures such as crowns and fixed bridges, and more of the profitable, low-overhead procedures, such as extractions and low-quality removable appliances.

Capitation schemes might be workable if the patient were first required to bring his mouth condition up to acceptable standards of dental health before entering the program, so that no great initial costs would accrue to the participating dentist, and if the patient were made equally responsible, for example, if penalties were assessed for missed appointments or for poor oral hygiene.

MEDICAID

Medicaid is a large-scale government-sponsored program through which a participating state pays the practitioner for treatment performed on community members deemed "medically indigent." Funds for this program come from federal, state, and local sources, the pattern varying from state to state. Payments are made on the fee-for-service unit-fee scale, a serious drawback, since reasonable fees cannot be maintained in the face of the widespread low-quality treatment common among Medicaid providers.

The experience of dentistry under Great Britain's national health service provides an example. Prior to national health service there were two classes of dentists working in England. One of these classes was university trained; the other learned the profession in apprentice fashion. The latter were known as "blood-and-vulcanite" dentists, because they generally merely extracted teeth and made dentures (vulcanite was a rubber-based material used in the past to make false teeth). Under the national health service's unit-fee system, the blood-and-vulcanite dentists made huge profits since they never bothered with the less-profitable service of *restoring* teeth. As their rising incomes were noticed, the response of the bureaucracy was characteristic: Reduce the fees across the board! And so the trained, conscientious dentists, already hard-pressed by the low earnings afforded by restoring teeth, now found fees so low that good dentistry could be done only at a loss. Thus, under economic pressure, the methods of the blood-and-vulcanite dentists were widely adopted, one of the reasons that the English have the highest incidence of false teeth in the world.

The American experience with Medicaid is similarly instructive. Some thirty years ago, when officials began the dental Medicaid program in New York, they consulted the local dental society for suggestions on how to ensure a high-quality program. They were told, reasonably enough, that you cannot have high quality without adequate fees, and following this advice the program originally set very generous fees, for example, allowing $5 a surface for an amalgam filling. This was generous, indeed; at the time the average good dentist was charging about $3.50 for a surface, while Dr. Poorwork was charging about a 50¢ for his botch of the job. It was expected that Poorwork would upgrade his work now that he was getting a fair fee. But the absence of quality controls led to disaster. The liberal fees enabled conscientious dentists to continue to provide an excellent service, but the low-quality dentist, instead of upgrading his service, grasped the opportunity to accept a great deal more profit from doing the same dreadful level of work. Dr. Poorwork was now simply taking $5 for his 50¢ filling. Some time later the bureaucrats, when they audited the program and found that some dentists who previously were making $7,000 a year were now making $70,000 through Medicaid, took typical action. They cut the fees! And so, once again, the bad dentists drove the good dentists from the system. This put Dr. Goodwork out of the program, while Dr. Poorwork, though making less, still cleaned up. A reasonable program of quality assurance would have avoided this disaster. At the present time, Medicaid fees are so low that it is impossible to produce high-quality dentistry under this system and make a living. Today Medicaid dentists generally find it virtually impossible to make a profit on dental Medicaid without resorting to hasty, sloppy work, falsifying records, inflating claims, and overtreatment.

For many years forensic experts have used dental records to identify people or dead bodies. But now the false reporting of dental records for claims has become so widespread that some leading forensic experts no longer consider dental records to be reliable enough for legal forensics!

MANAGED CARE: THE GREAT DECEPTION

Reformers, appalled by the runaway costs of our health care system, have advanced what they call managed care as a remedy. This merely means that third-party plans will establish parameters for care and costs, the idea being that better management will result in more efficient utilization. Managed care partisans claim that eliminating the fat, the wasted time, the duplication of effort, and the bureaucratic boondoggles will allow for significant savings.

We hear the word "efficiency" emphasized, implying that if the same amount of care is produced at less cost we are being more efficient. But there are other important measures of efficiency. *Long-term results* are a much better indicator. Paying less is worthless if what you are buying doesn't do the job, and in dentistry, only high-quality work does the job. To look for the cheap solution is simply throwing away money, at the same time condemning Americans to poor dental health.

But managed care in its present form is a deception. What is being managed is not the care provided but the cost of it. It is our contention that managed care cannot succeed unless it actually concerns itself with *care* as well as cost. For example, much publicity has been given to the notorious managed care rule that women who have just given birth leave the hospital the next day. Some new mothers are forced to go home despite suffering complications, a glaring example of how economic considerations can debase care. This problem is conspicuous in dentistry, where it is common for insurance consultants to inspect treatment plans and require inferior treatment to be done because of lower cost to the insurer.

Particularly appalling is the fact that many managed care plans are willing to cover fraudulent and quack treatments. As a gesture to the ignorance and gullibility of the public, some of these plans will pay for a variety of treatments that do not have scientific backing, from acupuncture and chiropractic to phony TMJ treatments. The insurers probably feel that if the quack treatments are denied, the patients will seek legitimate treatment, more effective but more expensive to the carrier. Perhaps the quacks will keep the patient tranquilized without having to pay for the genuinely effective but more expensive service of an honest doctor.

In dentistry particularly, managed care is a disaster. The cost managers have tried to lower costs by getting dentists to provide cheaper services, by hiring the "lowest bidder" providers. We will wind up with a system entirely staffed by Poorworks, ensuring the lowest level of dental quality which, as we have shown, is not only ruinous to the dental health of the public served by managed care but is also in the long run more expensive.

Costs are not reduced by wasting money on useless and damaging cheap care. The way to lower costs is to eliminate incompetence, quackery, overtreatment, and fraudulent reporting of work accomplished. In dentistry, the bottom-line mentality of managed care is leading to a situation where high-quality, appropriate dentistry will become a rare and expensive commodity. This is a shame, because the concept of managed care might, if used intelligently, *and if focused on quality care,* be a force in upgrading the quality and true efficiency of dental practice.

Today, many managed care plans are being formed around the principle of capitation (see above). The most noxious characteristic of managed care capitation plans is that they pit the interest of the doctor against the interest of the patient. In the typical capitation plan HMO, the doctor is given a set, limited money amount per patient; this amount is intended to cover the costs of treating the patient. Whatever is left over goes half to the HMO management and half to the doctor. The more treatment given to the patient, the more it costs and the less is left for the doctor. If treatment costs exceed the total amount left in that patient's treatment account, the doctor must make up the excess himself. Doctors are hesitant to refer patients to specialists, since the doctor, in effect, himself has to pay for the specialist.

Thus a powerful incentive is given the doctor to keep referrals and treatment costs to a minimum, thereby enriching the doctor and the entrepreneurs who run the HMO. Managed care HMOs are already showing immense profits. The chief executive officer of Foundation Health Corp. is compensated at more than $6,000,000 a year, while the CEO of U.S. Healthcare makes about $4,000,000. The enormous profits available explain why so many businessmen are eager to invest in the managed care field. And the shame of it all is that these profits are being generated by hasty and inadequate treatment to the patient, at the cost of the patient's health.

It should be noted here that managed care HMOs are shame-facedly attempting to keep their financial details from the public. Some doctors have told us that their contracts with managed care groups specify that the terms are to be kept secret! We can understand why; we would hate to stand in the way of an irate mob that has just learned that their doctors are being paid to *not* treat them.

OPTIONS

Single payer Rather than having, as Americans do, a great many sources of payment for health services, a single payer system concentrates financing of health care in a single authority, invariably the government. Its proponents claim that it will save huge sums through more efficient claims processing, eliminating most of the tons of paperwork currently generated by the thousands of third parties presently involved in our health system. This system is used for medical reimbursement in Canada. It does not address the problems of poor quality, inappropriate treatment, and fraudulent claims reporting, but with modification and quality assurance it may represent a workable scheme.

HMOs Health maintenance organizations usually compensate their doctors on a capitation plus bonus basis while enrolling patients with set membership fees. The bonuses come as a reward *not* to treat the patient (see above). Successful dental HMOs generally require patients before entering the program to bring their dental health up to a reasonably high level. Thus the program avoids being overwhelmed with the need to restore an avalanche of neglected mouths.

Referral plans In these schemes, patients are recruited and referred to a "participating" dentist. Patients usually pay an initiation fee that covers a few introductory services, usually an examination, X rays, and cleaning. The plan often promises that other work done by the plan dentist will be done at a discount (one plan advertises discounts up to 50 percent but does not specify 50 percent of what). Many of these plans require payments by the dentist to belong to the plan. At one time paying someone to send you patients was considered illegal as well as unethical, but apparently times have changed. One well-advertised scheme requires payments of many thousands of dollars every year by the participating dentists. Some of these plans claim that their dentists are monitored for quality, but other than the dentist having to prove he is licensed, we have seen no sign of any attempt at quality assurance.

Fee for service This is the way almost all American private dental practices operate. While at its best American dentistry sets the standard for the world, too many American dentists charge too much for poor-quality work. The flaws in fee for service have been shown in greater detail above.

Third-party financing This involves the introduction of a third party (usually an insurance carrier, acting for a union or other insured group) who will pay all or part of the doctor's fee. The impact of third-party payment is felt to some degree by almost every American dental practice. Commercial insurance companies account for 70 percent of American dental coverage, but no meaningful systems of quality assurance have been instituted.

RECOMMENDATIONS

Quality control This is essential. A program cannot succeed in its goals without quality assurance. The nature of dentistry makes it possible to institute workable quality controls at little expense and without great intrusions into dental offices. Computer programs can be set up to survey claims and track items such as tooth mortality, longevity of restorations, and efficiency of diagnostic procedures. X rays can be called for, which will show quality of restorations and comment on diagnoses. And occasional in-office inspections can reinforce the quality control procedure.

Through quality controls, the influence of insurance programs can have a powerful positive effect on the quality and cost of care. Quality assurance can weed out the frauds and decline payment and penalize doctors for incompetent or quack care. We believe that nationwide quality of dental care will take a dramatic turn for the better in the wake of quality controls.

Patient involvement The patient should be required to play an effective role in his oral health. Coverage can be reduced or eliminated for those who do not keep periodic diagnostic and preventive appointments and/or do not practice reasonable oral hygiene. Penalties should be assessed for time-wasting missed appointments.

Group practice It is expensive to practice and provide good dentistry. It is much more efficient to practice in a group, sharing certain major expenses as well as professional expertise and encouragement. It would seem important for each dentist to have a personal financial stake in the group, other than just salary, for incentives. Laws and tax policies could be drafted to encourage the formation of group practices.

Fee reform As we have shown above, the unit-fee-for-service system provides strong incentives toward low-quality service. We recommend that fee for service be replaced with a time-based system of compensation. A participating dentist would calculate his overhead and file a general fee per time with the insurer. His claims forms would list the procedures performed and the total time spent with the patient; payment would be made on that basis. Procedures requiring additional overhead, such as lab fees, would be compensated accordingly. Processing such claims would be much simpler, and the insurer would not suffer the long-range excess costs of Poorwork dentistry. Time-based fees are more rational, provide incentives for high-quality work, and simplify the paperwork of claims reporting. Insurance programs that incorporate effective quality controls would do well to promote the adoption of time-based fees. However, since time-based fees are also subject to abuses such as malingering and overreporting treatment time, quality controls must be designed to check efficiency and performance as well as quality of service.

Stop Rewarding Quackery Insurance carriers lose considerable sums to the quacks, whose fees the law requires them to pay. If the carriers can be made to understand that they can avoid paying these fees, they are likely to take action. One way might be to establish treatment classifications, as follows:

Category 1: Treatments considered safe, effective and legitimate. This would include conventional preventive and restorative dental treatments that have stood the test of time.

Category 2: Treatments that are experimental, not yet proven. These would include paste-filler endodontics, halitosis treatments, novel periodontal therapies, etc. To be considered ethical, experiments should be clearly labeled as experiments.

Category 3: Unproven or disproven treatments outside the parameters of accepted scientific practice (quackery).

Insurance policies could specifically deny coverage or payment for treatments in categories 2 and 3. Such provisions could save lots of money and also go far to halt the escalation of dental malpractice premiums and premiums for legitimate dental consumer coverage. (It is ironic that good dentists are subsidizing the bad dentists when it comes to malpractice insurance.)

The question arises: Who will make these category determinations, and under what criteria? This should present little difficulty since these differentiations have for the most part already been made by the dental schools and responsible dental scientists. We would hope that the American Dental Association will be responsible enough to participate in these evaluations. Publicizing these classifications through strong and effective consumer education, utilizing the media, could be the most potent deterrent against quackery.

We further suggest that legislation be enacted to make it compulsory that any health professional planning to use a category 2 or 3 treatment (experimental or nonscientific) make this clear to the patient and receive a written informed consent. While we would not want to restrict the right of any practitioner to treat patients as he sees fit, it is essential that the patient be clearly informed about the nature and scientific status of the planned treatment.

The use of these classifications can greatly assist the consumer in choosing offered treatment. In a free society the consumer does not have real freedom of choice if he is denied essential information. The potential buyer of an automobile does not have a free choice if he is not told the make, model, type, age, and condition of the car. Similarly, the consumer of health services cannot make a free choice if he is misinformed about the quality and scientific status of the proposed treatment. But if treatments are classified in this manner, and required to be so labeled, the consumer will then, finally, have a real, informed choice.

22. Quality Assurance

*

More than 40 percent of Americans have dental insurance. Many assume that this has led to an overall improvement in dental health. American dental health has indeed improved, but this is mostly because of fluoridation, better diet, and better awareness of oral hygiene. The availability of dental insurance has played a lesser part.

Insurance plans ostensibly provide adequate care to more people at less cost. They are supposed to be the answer to the horrendous boondoggle that our modern health care delivery system has become. But without quality assurance these plans are doomed to failure.

The absence of quality assurance is the major problem in virtually all dental insurance reimbursement programs, whether HMOs, managed care plans, or open or closed panels. Insurers and managed care plans do not screen out low-skilled and fraudulent dentists, who are often major providers for these plans. In the absence of workable quality controls, any insurance program will be abused and will fail to deliver a reasonable level of service at reasonable cost. Reimbursement programs that provide exactly the same compensation for work of widely varying quality inevitably sink to the lowest common denominator of care. This is because of the powerful incentive to do poor work built into such a reimbursement scheme. The hastiest and poorest service is, of course, the least expensive to provide and allows the most profit to the provider. Again we encounter the dismal paradox: The poorer the quality of service, the greater reward to the provider. In a free economy that is driven by economic reward, this spells death to good dentistry.

To form an analogy, suppose a program is set up to provide automobiles. The reimbursement scheme allows the same compensation to the provider whether the car provided is a new luxury vehicle or a battered old jalopy. Obviously, everyone will wind up with the jalopy. Yet every fee-for-service dental insurance program we know of operates (and fails) in this very fashion, allowing, for example, the same compensation for a "filling" whether the filling is the careful and meticulous restoration characteristic of good dentistry or the hasty and sloppy botch provided by low-quality volume dentists.

Right now there seems to be an epidemic of low-quality, inappropriate, and scientifically unsupported (quack) dental care. Compounding the fiasco is the widespread fraudulent reporting of claimed services. Added up, these factors result in dental disasters to the patients and massive unjustified and unnecessary expense for the carriers. Yet insurance carriers continue to pay for these procedures and for this fraud because they are not willing to institute a workable program of quality assurance and because they are afraid to face litigation.

Many patients have asked us to fill out insurance forms fraudulently. Insurance companies are often seen as fair game for fraud because "they're so wealthy." The insurance companies foster this adversarial relationship by setting up rules and regulations that make it difficult to get reimbursement even for legitimate claims. In many cases the claim instructions are so involved that courses have been developed to teach doctors how to fill out forms in order for their patients to get appropriate coverage. But there are courses of a darker character also being given, courses that instruct doctors how to generate insurance returns for treatment that is not covered.

Promotors of the TMJ quackery have made blunt recommendations to dentists to fool insurance companies into paying for their questionable treatments. Dentists have been told first to find out what treatments the insurance policy will pay for and then claim that these were the treatments done. If the patient is insured for medical procedures, then the dentist is advised to list his TMJ quackery as medical treatment. If the policy covers only dental treatment, the dentist should call if a dental procedure. If there is dual coverage, the dentist should apply for both. These bald-faced recommendations for fraud reflect the moral standard established by the original phony TMJ claims. (See Chapter 20.)

Here is an exact passage taken from an article some years back in a dental journal advising how to submit a TMJ claim. Rarely have we seen such a candid exhortation to fraud:

A. Strategy: Dental vs. Medical

1. If the patient's dental coverage pays for orthodontics and you handle the problem through this procedure, make no mention of orthopedics or temporomandibular joint therapy. Use the dental form.

2. If medical coverage—subscribe to orthopedics, neuromuscular pain, myofascial pain and do not use orthodontic terminology that would make your treatment a dental procedure. Use the medical procedure form.

3. Dual coverage—send the code procedure and "A" forms to the medical insurance carrier and the orthodontics forms to the dental insurance carrier.

4. First of all call the major medical insurance company to ask if they cover TMJ therapy. If they do not, submit procedure codes with no mention of TMJ.

The law adds a confounding factor. If a patient is denied coverage for a quack or fraudulent service, the patient is likely to sue, and, although the insurance carrier on its merits will always win such a case, the carrier usually feels it is cheaper to give in and pay for the fraud than to pay the costs of a legal action. And then there is always the chance that a scientifically illiterate jury will award a huge judgment in favor of the fraud.

In the face of the escalating expense caused by these factors, insurance carriers have been maintaining their profits by reducing compensation to participating dentists, increasing premiums and co-payment requirements for patients, and decreasing the number of covered services. These measures further debase the quality and effectiveness of the program and produce significant hardships on those dentists and patients who deliver and desire quality care. If the carriers instituted intelligent quality assurance mechanisms, this would upgrade the general quality of the program, eliminate abuse, be more profitable to the insurer, and provide a superior health service to the public.

Virtually every dental practice in the country has patients covered by insurance, and many dental practices rely heavily on third-party reimbursement schemes. As a result, the insurance industry has, in essence and in various degrees, become a major "employer" to many dentists and can strongly influence the choice of treatment options and the quality of care. The way things are now, this has usually worked to the detriment of the patient while simultaneously providing an opportunity for the insurance industry to be a powerful *positive* force on the American dental industry. With the establishing of quality criteria and treatment standards, and the effective implementation of quality controls, the insurance industry can simply refuse to pay for substandard, inappropriate, unneeded, fraudulent, or quack services. The upgrading of general dental quality would be immediate. Even practices that rely very little on insurance will be affected by the publicity and public pressure generated by the new focus on quality and the subsequent education of the public.

Part V

*

Conclusions

23. The Ideal Practice: Recommendations

*

American dentistry at its best is the world's standard and can accomplish almost miraculous results. The best American dentistry can in nearly every case succeed in enabling a cooperating patient to maintain healthy, functioning teeth for a lifetime. But the reality is that most people are missing many or all of their teeth by the time they reach old age, and this includes not just people who have neglected their teeth but also people who have gone to the dentist routinely. How can we reconcile the statement lauding the excellence of American dentistry with the dismal results we see? The answer is that the quality of dental service varies sharply among dentists, and only high-quality dentistry achieves these fine results.

From the standpoint of society, the purpose of the dental profession is to maintain the dental health of the population. Certain social engineers have proposed managed care concepts to efficiently meet this need. But, as we have shown, the managed care concept focuses only on reducing cost, not on improving or extending care. The word "efficiency" is emphasized, as if to say that the same amount of care produced at less cost equals efficiency. But there are better ways to evaluate efficiency than immediate cost per procedure; factoring in long-term results will provide a more intelligent assessment. (See Chapter 21.)

It is our contention that all American dentists can work at the high level necessary to produce excellent results. All graduates of American dental schools who are licensed to practice here have demonstrated the ability to produce high-level results; they have passed school and licensing examinations to prove this. But the conditions of practice imposed on most dentists compromise their ability to produce quality results. We believe that dental practices throughout the country should be redesigned to allow the best dentistry to be produced.

The first consideration should be for working conditions that will allow the dentist and his auxiliaries to perform their duties in comfort and without undue strain. The performance of good dentistry is difficult enough without having to overcome poor equipment, discomfort, and fatigue. Dentistry, perhaps more than the other medical professions, is demanding mentally *and* physically. The economic problems of a general dentist are daunting, and to meet overhead and make a living he generally has to work a week of full days. After spending seven or eight hours of intense mental concentration combined with arduous physical strain, a dentist knows he has done a day's work. And this is even worse for the good dentist, whose work is so much more exacting. Any social effort directed at solving the country's dental need must consider the working conditions of our dentists. Dentistry is a tough job, which should be made easier. The designing of an efficient practice environment must never overlook this.

GROUP PRACTICE: A MAJOR SOLUTION

For generations the typical dentist practiced by himself in his own private office. As a rugged individualist, his freedom, professional as well as personal, was complete. He was entirely on his own when it came to prescribing treatment for patients; he wasn't compelled to submit his planned treatment to any bureaucratic panel for approval. His decisions for patient treatment options were his own, limited only perhaps to what the patient could afford. He was the only and final authority on the competence and appropriateness of his treatment. His freedom extended in other directions: He could make his own schedule, plan vacations, work hard or leisurely as he wished. Only economic pressure imposed limitations on these freedoms of solo practice.

He was also free, depending on his conscience and the local economic climate, to practice good dentistry or become a Poorwork, a fraud, or a quack.

Group practice diminishes these freedoms. Daily scheduling, vacations, working hours, leisure time, and level of quality all must conform to the collective requirements of the group. Despite this, we feel that the enormous advantages of practicing with other professionals outweigh the freedom of movement afforded by solo practice. The solo dental office seems slowly to be on its way out. More and more group practices are being formed, and most newly graduated dentists are going into group practice. It simply is too expensive to open an old-fashioned solo practice, nor is it a good idea to let the new and inexperienced graduate loose on the public. A hospital internship or a good-quality group practice is the best way for a new dentist to start in his profession.

In a good-quality group practice, a dentist whose work is seen daily by other good dentists is not going to relax into slipshod methods. Intimate contact with other professionals has a bolstering effect on one's own quality, particularly in the case of the new dental graduate, who benefits from the support and encouragement and help of the experienced dentists in the group. Improved treatment techniques will be introduced more quickly in the group environment. The group can include one or more specialists. A group of experienced dentists is in a position to evaluate the competence of a specialist, so a specialist in a good group is probably a good specialist. Furthermore, the group can utilize the services of auxiliaries, which considerably lightens the burdens of the member dentists.

But it is disappointing to have to say that most group practices today are not practicing high-quality dentistry. For the most part they have been formed to take advantage of burgeoning third-party schemes, Medicaid, union and company plans, and private insurers. They are also taking advantage of the economic plight of many young dentists who cannot afford to open a private practice and older dentists in economic difficulty because of the competition of closed-panel plans. (See Chapter 21.) They are hiring these dentists at relatively low salaries and impelling them to produce a lot of quick, shoddy work. Since these plans generally pay the clinics on a fee-for-service basis (in other circumstances this is called "piecework"), the owners of the group would rather their dentists do three shoddy fillings in half an hour than one excellent job. That way they are paid three times as much despite the fact that the shoddy fillings are a poor service that will not last. They don't care; when the shoddy fillings fail, the insurers will pay for an extraction for the tooth and then for a cheap replacement, which in turn will fail. As long as compensation continues on a fee-for-service basis without quality controls, this travesty will endure.

Perhaps these problems can be overcome and compensation be structured to provide incentives for high-quality service. As we suggested earlier, a time-based fee system coupled with effective quality assurance may be the most workable and fairest method of compensation. The skill of a trained dentist is meaningless unless he has enough time to effectively use his skill. As we have emphasized, the critical factor in quality is time; therefore, we believe the dentist should be paid for the amount of time spent with the patient. We strongly recommend that a time-based system be universally adopted. We have used such a system successfully in our practice for more than twenty years.

We believe that, with adequate economic support and intelligent design and execution, a near-perfect system of group dental practice can be effected. It goes without saying that the efficient, high-quality practice of the future must, first of all, have the plant and the facilities to provide the environment needed for successful practice. Modern equipment for the efficient practice of the best dentistry must be combined with facilities to meet and maintain hygienic standards and to attend to record-keeping and the business end of the practice. Offices must be sufficient in size and furnishings to provide comfortable conditions for patients and practitioners. These conditions are a given. But most important are the personnel and how they are used. Much of this depends on economics. If the financial structure of the group is satisfactory to its members, then the group can function to provide a decent service to patients while keeping the personnel, professional as well as auxiliaries, satisfied. And this means allowing the personnel enough in the way of compensation while not overworking them.

24. Parting Shots

*

We've tried to provide enough information so that anyone confronted with a dilemma concerning dentistry can make a sensible and informed decision. This applies to the dental consumer, insurance executive, government or union official, HMO entrepreneur, dental student, or dentist. We would like to reiterate some of the more pertinent points we have emphasized.

To the Consumer

Remember, in looking for quality dental service, the most important element is *time*. No matter what kind of dental facility you use, if not enough time is given for your treatment, the treatment will be substandard. A crowded waiting room from which patients come and go every few minutes is *a bad sign*.

If a dentist tells you something that doesn't sound right, for example, that you need a tremendous number of expensive crowns that you never suspected, or if you suddenly need full-mouth gum surgery, *ask him to write it down and sign it*. A doctor of integrity is always willing to put what he thinks in writing and sign it. The quack or fraud, if pressed, wants to deny ever making such statements and, of course, will not sign anything put in writing.

When you sign an insurance form, look it over carefully. Don't permit a dentist to report treatment that wasn't done.

Be alert for signs of quackery. Be skeptical about what you see and hear on TV and radio and in the press. Don't be a sucker. Your best bet is to learn the techniques of critical scientific thinking. Join the National Council Against Health Fraud, P.O. Box 1276, Loma Linda, CA 92354. If you think you've been victimized by a fraudulent or quack dentist, you can contact the Victim Redress Committee of the council for help.

To the Dental Educator

Make sure that dental students are given courses in scientific critical thinking. It's probable that most dental quacks sincerely believe their own aberrant theories. A knowledge of scientific thinking techniques would cure them. Courses on ethics should also be required.

To the Union Member or Plain Citizen Joining a Plan

Make sure the plan is not simply cheap but also allows the dentist to spend sufficient time to do his job right and provides for quality assurance checks.

To the Government or Union Official

High-quality dentistry requires constant intense concentration and is physically as well as mentally demanding. If you truly want a well-working quality plan, make sure your dentist employees have enough time to do their work, enjoy pleasant working conditions, have a staff of well-trained and competent auxiliaries, have enough time off, and get paid well.

To the Insurance Executive

You have a unique opportunity to correct most of the abuses and shortcomings of the medical delivery system without turning the whole system upside down. Simply institute in your programs an effective system of quality assurance and crack down on quackery and fraud. Refuse to pay for incompetent work or quackery and penalize fraudulent behavior. If you are serious about this, and are willing to do what it takes, you'll save enough to rehabilitate the whole system, and you will sharply upgrade the quality of health service almost overnight. The opportunity is here to change the incentive of managed care from the poorer the service, the greater the reward, to the better the service, the greater the reward.

To Licensing Boards and Legislators

Don't be fooled by charismatic quacks who want you to mandate insurance payments for their quackery. Study scientific critical thinking in order to make more sensible decisions. And once you better understand quackery and fraud, take powerful steps to discipline and punish and eliminate the quacks and the frauds.

To Organized Dentistry

Make some meaningful attempts to set scientific standards and ensure the quality of postgraduate courses given to dentists. End the shameful practice of allowing courses in pseudoscience and quackery to be given under the sponsorship of organized dentistry.

Stop putting up with Dr. Poorwork. Help improve the economic climate of the profession. Publish and publicize criteria of competent practice. We have suggested the following classification of dental procedures: (1) generally safe and effective; (2) experimental; and (3) unsound or disproven (quackery). If such a classification were adopted, insurance companies would have a basis for refusing to pay treatments in categories 2 and 3, and dentists would hesitate to use questionable therapies.

Glossary

abrasion. The wearing away of tooth structure usually caused by using a hard toothbrush and improper brushing technique.

abscess. A localized, walled-off infection. A *tooth abscess* is caused by bacteria getting into the pulp (nerve) of the tooth. A *periodontal abscess* is caused by an infection between the gum and the tooth.

abutment. The tooth or teeth that act as anchors for a fixed or removable bridge.

acrylic. A plastic used to make dentures, false teeth, and veneers.

air abrasion. A revival of an old technique, using a sandblaster type of device, for preparing teeth for fillings. The safety and usefulness of this machine have not been established.

allergy. A specific biological and physiological response by a susceptible person to a particular substance.

alveolar bone. The jawbone that is immediately adjacent to the roots of the teeth.

alveolectomy. The surgical removal of jawbone in order to smooth irregularities that might interfere with the function of dentures.

amalgam. The most common and for most purposes the best filling material for back teeth. It is also known as silver amalgam because it is a mixture of mercury with silver, tin, copper, and zinc.

analgesia. The partial loss of pain perception. In dentistry this usually refers to the use of nitrous oxide (laughing gas) to produce a state of incomplete anesthesia; the patient, although conscious, has a lowered awareness of pain and is more relaxed.

anesthesia. The absence of pain perception. A dental patient usually receives *local anesthesia,* an injection near the tooth; the tooth and gum are numb but the patient is totally awake. With *general anesthesia,* the patient is unconscious.

anterior teeth. The six upper and six lower front teeth: two eye-teeth (canines), two lateral incisors, and two central incisors (front teeth).

antibiotic. A drug that kills, weakens, or slows the reproduction of germs.

ANUG. Acute necrotizing ulcerative gingivitis, also known as trench mouth or Vincent's disease.

apex. The tip of the root.

apicoectomy. The surgical removal of the apex of a root together with any surrounding infection.

arch. The shape the teeth have in the mouth. There is an upper dental arch and a lower arch.

auxiliaries. The people who assist the dentist, including dental assistants, lab technicians, and dental hygienists.

baby teeth. The popular name for the first teeth, also called *deciduous* or *primary teeth*. There are normally twenty baby teeth.

base. An insulating cement placed under a filling or crown to lessen sensitivity to heat and cold and to prevent damage from the filling material.

biopsy. A diagnostic test in which a small piece of tissue is surgically removed so that it can be examined by a pathologist (a specialist in diagnosing disease) under a microscope.

bite. The way the upper and lower teeth fit together when the jaws are closed. Also called *occlusion*.

black hairy tongue. A condition in which fungi that normally live in the mouth grow excessively because of the routine use of hydrogen peroxide mouth rinses or antibiotic therapy.

block injection. The anesthetizing of a defined area by "blocking" the major nerve branch to that area. Usually used for the lower teeth, resulting in the lip, teeth, and tongue of half the lower jaw getting numb. Compare *infiltration*.

bonding. A technique for attaching restorative materials to tooth structure. Also the term giving to the cosmetic repair or veneering of a tooth, usually a front tooth.

bone loss. The shrinking of jawbone support around the root of a tooth. This is the major characteristic of gum disease.

bone resorption. The process by which the alveolar (jaw) bone is lost. During orthodontics this process is controlled by the dentist, so that bone is lost in the direction the tooth is being moved and replaced behind the tooth. This is how the orthodontist seemingly moves the tooth through "solid bone."

braces. The lay term for *orthodontic appliances*. They reposition the teeth.

bridge. The general term for a restoration that replaces missing teeth. A *removable bridge* can be removed from the mouth for cleaning. A *fixed bridge* cannot be removed.

bruxism. Grinding the teeth, usually while sleeping. It appears to be hereditary.

bruxomania. Grinding the teeth while awake.

calcium. One of the essential minerals necessary for healthy teeth and bones, as well as proper nerve function.

calculus. The hard yellow to brown residue (also known as *tartar*) that forms on teeth at the gum line due to incomplete or improper home care.

canker sore. A small whitish ulcer that appears in the mouth. It is related to a cold sore and lasts ten to fourteen days.

cantilever bridge. A fixed bridge that is supported only on one side with the false tooth hanging off the end.

cap. Lay term for *crown*.

caries. The scientific term for tooth decay.

casting. A restoration that is cast in metal outside of the mouth and then cemented or placed in the mouth. Metal crowns, inlays, and partial dentures are usually made with castings.

cast post. See *post.*

Cavitron. A device that scales and cleans the teeth with an ultrasonic handpiece.

cavity. A defect in a tooth that is usually caused by caries.

cellulitis. A massive, potentially dangerous swelling caused by uncontrolled infection. A dentist or physician should be seen immediately.

cementum. The hard tissue that covers the root of a tooth.

charting. An examination of the depth of the periodontal pockets.

clasp. The "hook" or "clip" that helps to hold a removable partial denture in place. Clasps are usually made of metal, but they can be plastic.

cleaning. See *prophylaxis.*

composite. A mixture of a plastic binder with particles of much harder material such as glass or ceramic. Composites may be either chemically or light cured (hardened) and are the materials most commonly used when a tooth is bonded.

compound. A hard, resinous wax that is used to take impressions. It is a thermoplastic material that gets soft when heated.

copper band. A technique for taking an impression of a tooth. A cylinder of copper is fitted to the tooth and an impression material such as compound is put in the band and pressed over the tooth preparation. When the impression material sets, the band is removed and a duplicate of the prepared tooth is made from the impression.

crown. The part of the tooth, covered with enamel, that is above the gum. A synthetic replacement of all of the enamel is also called a crown.

curettage. The removal of the dead inner lining of the gum in a periodontal pocket. It is often performed with local anesthesia, and the calculus is removed at the same time.

cyst. A fluid-filled sac within the body. An oral cyst is detectable on an X ray.

decay. *Caries.*

deciduous teeth. The scientific name for *baby teeth.*

dental floss. The thin "string" that is passed gently between the teeth to remove food particles and plaque.

dentin. The hard, bonelike tissue that makes up the inner core of a tooth. Dentin is "living" tissue, which explains why a deep cavity hurts.

dentist. "A prestidigitator, who, putting metal into your mouth, pulls coins out of your pocket." Ambrose Bierce used this definition in *The Devil's Dictionary.* There are other definitions of this word, some more kind.

dentition. The teeth and their arrangement.

denture adhesive. A sticky gumlike material that helps hold dentures in place.

dentures. The common term for removable false teeth. A *partial denture* replaces some of the teeth; a *full denture* replaces all of the teeth.

denturism. The movement to legalize the making and selling of dentures by non-dentists.

diastema. A gap between the teeth, usually the upper front teeth.

die. The exact duplicate of a tooth that is used to fabricate a cast restoration.

enamel. The hard light-yellow tissue that covers the crown of a tooth. It is second only to diamond as the hardest naturally occurring substance, but its crystallike structure can be fractured.

endodontics. The study of the pulp (nerve) and its treatment.

eruption. The process by which the teeth grow through the gums and assume their position in the mouth.

exodontia. The extraction of teeth.

explorer. The sharp-pointed curved instrument that is used to examine the surfaces of the teeth for decay, cracks, and calculus and to see if a restoration fits properly. Often called the "pick" by patients.

extraction. The removal of a tooth from the mouth.

eyeteeth. The four corner upper and lower teeth. Also called *canines*.

facing. The visible, tooth-colored part of a restoration. Acrylic, composite plastic, or porcelain is used as facing.

filling. A restoration "filling" a defect, often a hole, in the tooth.

fistula. A narrow tunnel that conducts the pus from the site of an infection to another location. A fistula in the mouth is commonly called a *gum boil*.

fixed bridge. A tooth replacement that is supported by and cemented to some of the remaining teeth.

flap surgery. A type of periodontal surgery for extensive and deep pockets. The gums are loosened from the underlying bone and "flapped" back, and the defects in the bone and the exposed tooth structure meticulously cleaned. The flap is then sutured back into position, and a dressing is placed over the wound.

fluoridation. The addition of fluoride to drinking water to help prevent tooth decay. Most drinking water in the United States contains natural or added fluoride.

forceps. Plierlike instrument used to extract a tooth.

full denture. A removable denture that replaces all of the patient's teeth in one arch.

galvanic reaction. Pain caused by an electric current in the mouth between two different metallic restorations. This is not dangerous and almost always disappears within a few days.

general anesthesia. The production of an unconscious state by the use of drugs.

geographic tongue. A benign condition in which an area of the tongue loses its characteristic color and texture. The shape and location of this area can change with time. The condition is harmless and needs no treatment.

gingiva. The soft tissue surrounding the teeth; the gums.

gingivectomy. The surgical removal of gum tissue, often a part of periodontal therapy.

gingivitis. An inflammation of the gums and an early step in the development of periodontal disease.

gold foil. An antiquated method of filling using pure gold that is hammered into the prepared tooth.

grinding. See *bruxism* and *bruxomania.*

gum boil. A swelling on the gum caused by drainage from a deeper infection; a *fistula.*

halitosis. The term invented by advertising copywriters to describe bad mouth odor.

high. The lay term for a filling that interferes with the normal way the teeth fit together.

history. The complete medical and dental record of a patient.

hydrogen peroxide. A compound that releases oxygen. It is the active component in all dental bleaching systems and is also sometimes recommended, in a less concentrated form, as a mouthwash.

hyperemia. Sensitivity of the tooth to temperature (usually cold), and sweets. This can be the first step in the formation of an abscess.

immediate denture. A denture that can be placed immediately following the extraction of a patient's teeth.

impaction. A mature tooth that has not erupted all the way through the jawbone and gum.

implant. An artificial device that replaces the root of a tooth and can be used to anchor a new tooth or a bridge or denture.

impression. The first step in making a duplicate model of part of the patient's mouth.

incisors. The four upper and four lower front teeth. The two middle teeth are *central incisors;* the two on the sides are *lateral incisors.*

infiltration. Common method of anesthetizing upper teeth. Numbs only a small area around the tooth.

inlay. A filling made in the dental laboratory and later cemented or bonded to the tooth.

intraoral camera. A relatively new diagnostic device that employs a very small TV camera to view the tissues of the mouth with excellent lighting and magnification. The image can be studied by both the dentist and the patient; some of the equipment can even print out pictures of what is seen on the TV screen.

jacket. A full crown on a front tooth, normally made of porcelain.

Jerome mercury tester. An industrial device that some anti-amalgam dentists use to frighten patients into having perfectly good silver-amalgam fillings replaced.

laminate. A thin veneer of plastic or porcelain that is made in the lab and then bonded to a tooth. Laminates are usually used to correct cosmetic problems.

laughing gas. Nitrous oxide gas, so-called because during one of the stages of anesthesia the patient is apt to react with laughter.

local anesthesia. The technique that anesthetizes only a local area of the body with the patient remaining conscious. The most common form of anesthesia used by dentists.

longevity. How long a dental repair lasts.

malocclusion. Abnormal relationship of the upper to lower teeth.

managed care. General term for a system of reimbursement of health services designed to raise efficiency and reduce costs.

mandible. The lower, movable jaw.

margin. The border or boundary of a dental restoration with the tooth.

Maryland bridge. Also called a *resin-bonded bridge*. A semipermanent way of replacing missing teeth by bonding a framework with false teeth to some of the remaining teeth. Less expensive than conventional fixed bridge work but not as durable.

materia alba. The soft whitish debris that accumulates around the teeth, also called *plaque*.

maxilla. The upper jaw.

mercury. A heavy silvery metal that is liquid at room temperature, widely used in dental silver fillings.

milk teeth. Lay term for *deciduous* or *primary teeth*.

molars. The twelve back teeth, including wisdom teeth.

mouth mirror. The small mirror a dentist or hygienist uses to see areas of the mouth that are inaccessible to direct vision.

nerve. The lay term for the *pulp* of the tooth. "Killing the nerve" is an old-fashioned expression for root canal therapy.

night guard. A plastic appliance that covers all the upper or lower teeth and is used at night to prevent the wear of the teeth caused by grinding.

nitrous oxide. See *laughing gas*.

Novocain. One of the first local anesthetic drugs.

occlusion. The way the teeth on the upper and lower jaws come together; the *bite*.

onlay. A restoration made in the laboratory that covers the cusps of a tooth and is cemented or bonded.

oral cavity. The mouth.

oral hygiene. The cleansing of the mouth by brushing, flossing, rinsing, etc.

oral surgery. The specialty of dentistry that deals with operations on the oral cavity including extractions, cyst and tumor removal, cleft palate correction, fixing of broken jaws, rehabilitation after accidents and cancer surgery. Oral surgeons are also known as *maxillofacial surgeons*.

orthodontics. The specialty of dentistry that deals with correcting misalignment of the teeth both for cosmetic and functional reasons. The lay term for an orthodontic appliance is *braces*.

overdenture. A denture that fits over specially prepared roots or implants.

palliative treatment. Treatment to reduce emergency pain.

parasthesia. The loss of feeling to a part of the body. In dentistry this is usually a consequence of damage to one of the facial nerves during surgery, implant placement, or an overextended root canal filling. In many cases feeling will return, at least partially, after a period of time.

partial. A removable denture that replaces only some of the teeth.

pedodontics. The specialty of dentistry that deals with the treatment of children.

pericementitis. Inflammation around the root of a tooth causing pain when pressure is applied to the tooth.

periodontal disease. Disease of the gums and supporting tissues of the teeth.

periodontal probe. A thin calibrated instrument used to measure the depth of bone defects around the teeth caused by periodontal disease.

periodontics. The specialty of dentistry that deals with the diagnosis and treatment of periodontal disease.

permanent filling. The lay term for a filling that is designed to give long-term service.

permanent teeth. The adult teeth that replace the *deciduous* or *primary teeth*. There are thirty-two permanent teeth, sixteen in each arch.

pit. A tiny enamel defect, usually on the chewing surface of the molars (back teeth).

placebo. From the latin for "I shall please." A treatment that works because of the belief in the treatment rather than the content of the treatment.

plaque. The slimy combination of microorganisms, food debris, and mucus that adheres to the teeth and is thought to be the major contributor to gum disease and tooth decay.

pontic. The false tooth on a bridge.

porcelain fillings. The lay term for a white, tooth-colored filling. These fillings are usually made of plastic, but some inlays have been made of laboratory processed porcelain.

post. The metal strut that is placed into the root of a badly broken-down tooth after root canal therapy to increase the retention of a restoration, usually a crown. There are several kinds of posts. Prefabricated posts can be screwed into the root canal (screw posts), but can lead to root fractures. Posts can be cast to fit the canal and then cemented into place (cast posts). And prefabricated posts can be custom fitted and cast to a core, making a strong, durable one piece cemented post-core.

post-core. The post plus a partial replacement for the lost internal structure of the tooth. A crown is always cemented over a post-core.

post-crown. A one-piece post-core and crown.

posterior teeth. The *back teeth;* the *premolars* and *molars.*

premolar. The teeth in front of the molars.

primary teeth. The *deciduous* or *baby teeth.* There are twenty primary teeth, all of which will be replaced by the permanent teeth.

prognosis. The learned estimate of the prospects for success of a treatment.

prophylaxis. The cleaning (scaling) and polishing of the teeth.

prosthesis. An artifical device to replace missing parts of the body. In dentistry, a prothesis usually replaces teeth, but it may also replace parts of the oral structures lost to disease, birth defects, or accidents.

prosthodontics. The specialty that deals with replacing teeth with bridges and dentures.

pulp. The tissue inside a tooth made up of nerve tissue, blood vessels, and connective tissue.

pulp capping. A technique that covers a small area of exposed pulp tissue with a medicated filling material. A permanent filling is usually placed over the pulp cap.

pulp chamber. The part of the pulp found within the crown of the tooth. The pulp chamber is usually a large, open, hollow space in the tooth that connects with the thin, narrow pulp canals in the roots.

pulpectomy. The complete removal of the pulp, as is done in root canal therapy.

pulpitis. An inflammation of the pulp leading to sensitivity to temperature and pressure. The major cause of a toothache.

pulpotomy. The partial removal of the pulp.

pyorrhea. The old term for gum disease.

quackery. The promotion of medical schemes or remedies known to be false or of unproven benefits—for a profit.

rebase. The addition of acrylic (plastic) to a denture by a laboratory procedure.

rehabilitation. The restoration of a badly diseased mouth to good function and appearance.

reimplantation. The process of putting back a patient's own traumatically lost tooth or teeth.

reline. The addition of plastic to a denture, to make up for shrinkage of the underlying jawbone.

removable bridge. A tooth replacement that can be removed from the mouth for cleaning. Also known as a "partial."

restorations. The term for repairs to the teeth.

restorative dentistry. The area of dental practice that deals with restorations.

retained root. A root that has been left in the jaw after the tooth has been removed or knocked out.

root. The part of the tooth under the gums that anchors the tooth to the jaw. The root is not covered by enamel but by cementum.

root canal. The hollow tunnel-like area within the root that contains pulp tissue and connects the pulp chamber with the nerves and blood vessels in the jaw.

root canal therapy. The removal of the pulp and the filling of the remaining cleaned, shaped space (root canal) with a compacted material. *Endodontics.*

rubber dam. A soft latex sheet that is used to isolate and keep dry either a single tooth, as in root canal therapy, or several teeth, as when fillings are being done.

saliva. The scientific term for spit. Saliva contains enzymes, mucus, bacteria, viruses, and white blood cells.

saliva ejector. The curved device placed in the mouth by the dentist to remove saliva by suction.

salivary glands. The large glands in the cheek and under the tongue that produce saliva.

scaling. The careful and meticulous removal of plaque and calculus by the use of hand instruments.

screw post. See *post.*

sealants. Bonded plastics used to fill the grooves on the chewing surface of permanent molars to prevent decay.

secondary dentin. Dentin the pulp of the tooth produces in response to irritation.

silver fillings. Fillings made of silver amalgam.

space maintainer. A device that holds the space for a permanent tooth when a primary (baby) tooth is lost prematurely.

splinting. Attaching two or more teeth together so they act as one stronger unit. The teeth are normally splinted with crowns, but they can also be bonded together with composite plastic or metal restorative materials.

supernumery tooth. An extra tooth.

supporting tissues. The gingiva (gums), periodontal ligament, and the jawbone, which support the teeth.

surface. One of the five faces of a tooth. Most dentists and insurance plans base the amount they charge or pay on the number of surfaces that are restored.

tartar. The lay term for *calculus*.

temporary filling. A filling, usually medicated, used for a short time to protect the tooth until a permanent restoration can be made.

TMJ. The temporomandibular joint, which connects the lower movable jaw to the upper stationary jaw. Also the popular name for a set of disorders and conditions with the common symptoms of facial pain and/or restriction of opening and movement.

third-party provider. An agency that pays part or all of the dental bill but is not involved in the actual treatment. Insurance companies, unions, and government agencies are common third parties.

tooth bud. The embryonic structure within the jawbone that will develop into a tooth.

torus. A harmless bony growth on the palate or on the inside of the lower jaw.

transplant. The insertion of a natural tooth into the socket of another tooth.

trauma. Injury produced by accident, violence, severe temperature change, chemicals, etc. Occlusal trauma is caused by improper tooth alignment.

trench mouth. See *ANUG*.

unerupted tooth. A tooth that has not grown into its proper place in the mouth.

veneer. The aesthetic facing on a crown or a facing bonded directly to the tooth. A preformed veneer made of plastic or porcelain bonded to the tooth is called a *laminate*.

wisdom teeth. The third molars, which erupt between the ages of eighteen and twenty-five and can cause discomfort.

xerostomia. Decrease in saliva.

Index